A Parent's Handbook of

EVERYDAY LIFE SKILLS for AUTISTIC CHILDREN

Lesley Burton

A Parent's Handbook of
EVERYDAY LIFE SKILLS
for AUTISTIC CHILDREN

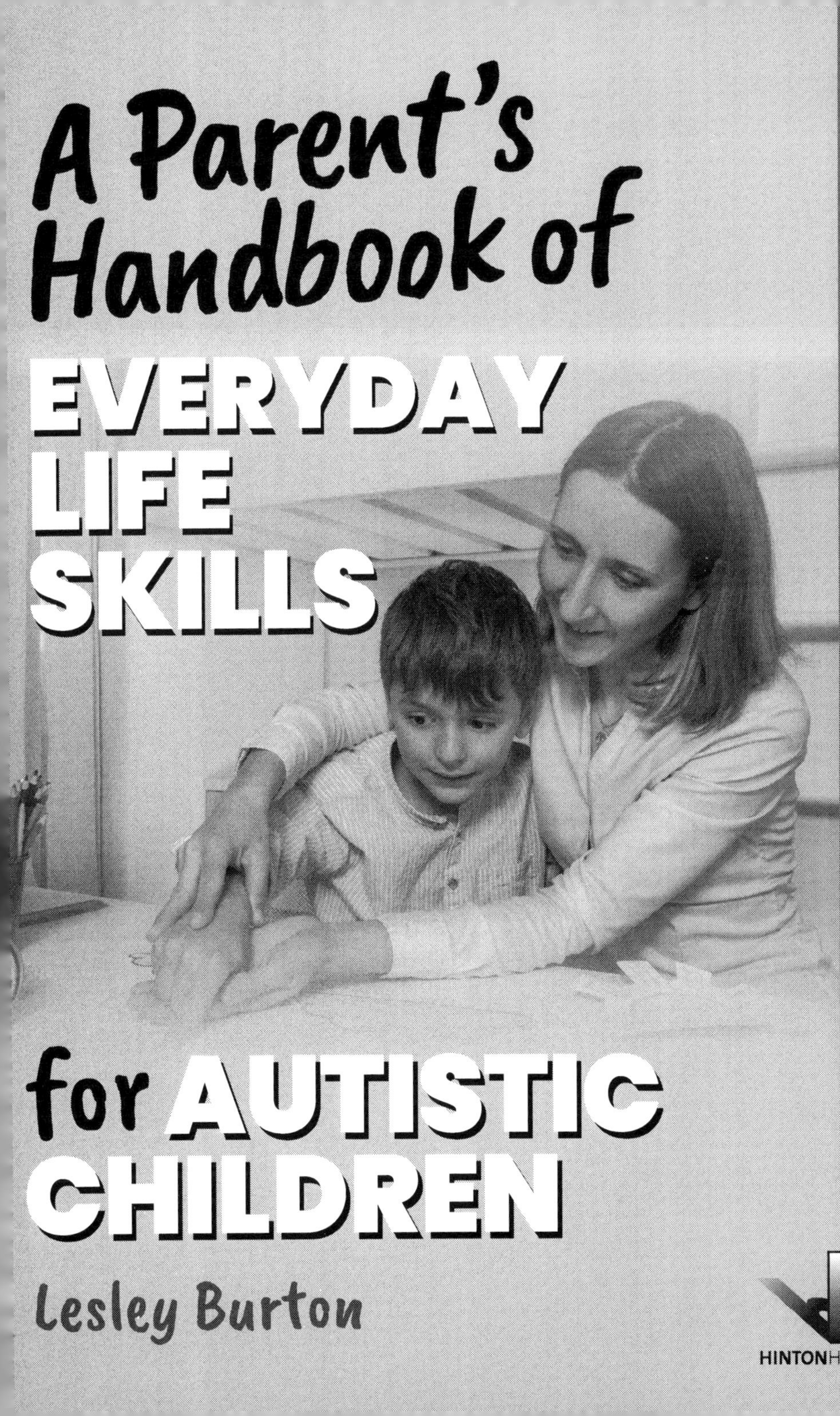

Lesley Burton

HINTON HOUSE Parenting

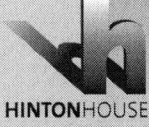

HINTON HOUSE

First published in 2022 by
Hinton House Publishers Ltd
T +44 (0)1280 822557 E info@hintonpublishers.com

www.hintonpublishers.com

British Library Cataloguing in Publication Data

A CIP catalogue record for this book is available from the British Library.

ISBN 978 1 912112 96 8

Printed and bound in the United Kingdom

Contents

About Lesley Burton

I trained as a chartered secretary and live and work in London. I have three children; my eldest son had glue ear and a language delay and my second son, Eddie, has autism spectrum disorder (ASD). I also have a younger daughter. In 2005, having spent many, many hours in speech therapy with my boys, and after attending the National Autistic Society EarlyBird programme, which I accessed through our local child development team, I decided to set up an online shop selling toys for children with special needs, specialising in resources to support communication and interaction. This gave me marvellous access to lots of wonderful and autism-friendly resources, which I could make available to parents, nurseries, schools and therapists. I also met many amazing parents dedicating their lives to helping their children, mostly with ASD, through parents' group events, exhibitions and conferences.

I sold the toy business in 2020 to concentrate on creating a blog, writing this book and speaking at events.

Further information available at: www.eddiesmum.com

About Eddie

Eddie was diagnosed with ASD at the age of 2 years 6 months, learned to use PECS (picture exchange communication system) at 2 years 8 months, and started in the nursery of a special school aged three. He has attended special schools providing autistic specialist provision for all his educational life. He was totally non-verbal until the age of nine, when his first word was 'No' and his second word was 'Yeah'.

He now has an increased vocabulary but can't speak clearly enough for all to understand him, which is a source of frustration for him and makes him very anxious as well as vulnerable. He has many sensory issues, and some challenging behaviour, and only likes a narrow, but reasonably healthy, range of foods.

Eddie has very little understanding of the world around him and has no friends of his own age, except those in his class at school. He could never have a tooth extraction, give a blood sample, stay at home alone or travel independently. He clearly loves his family and carers, but his toy Pingu is his best friend whom he confides in.

Eddie sleeps well at night and wakes up every morning cheerful and full of enthusiasm; he looks forward months ahead to holidays, especially in familiar places. He keeps himself busy and happily amused when on his own, playing with toys and computer games, so long as his devices and the Wi-Fi work. There are also plenty of activities he enjoys, such as tenpin bowling, crazy golf, going to the gym, making cupcakes, and going to a farm and nursery where he helps with gardening and looking after the animals.

He is both a joy and an inspiration on a daily basis. Having a child with autism is very challenging, but it is also very grounding: it brings a totally unique dimension to your family life, through the experiences of caring for your child and learning to see things in a very different way.

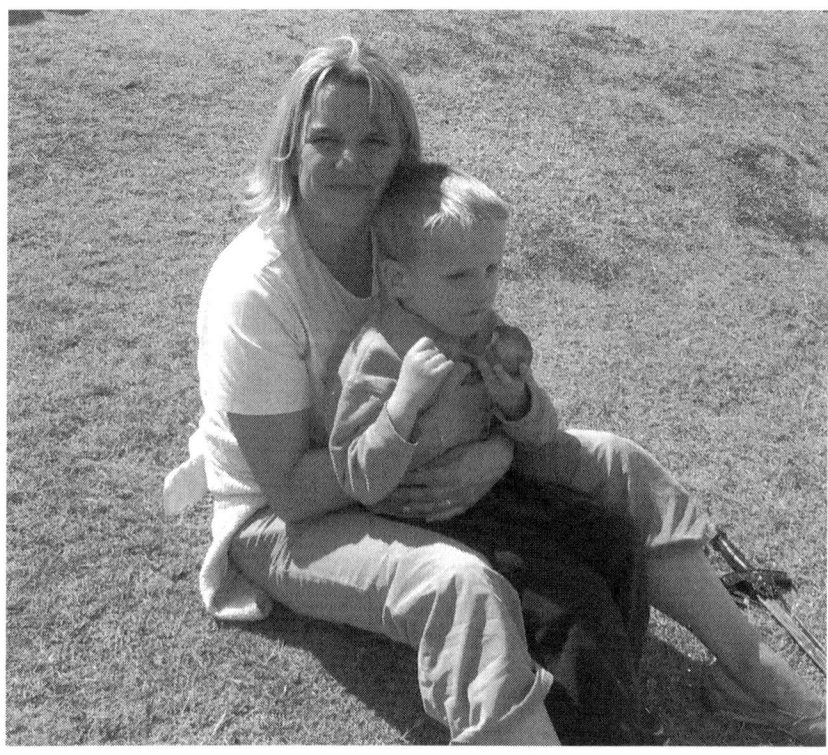

Eddie and Lesley in the early days

Foreword

I started to do a few talks at parent groups and childminder training days, and at The Autism Show (an annual national event that takes place in London, Manchester and Birmingham), about the joys and challenges of having an autistic child in our family. These were so well received, and there was such an appetite for hearing about our experiences, that I decided to write a book that could be helpful to others in the same position.

Through my toy business, I met so many parents like me, struggling with day-to-day issues, that I felt I should share the wealth of knowledge I have amassed over the last 21 years. I have gathered, in this accessible book, the strategies that we have found useful for our autistic son, Eddie. I like to imagine that this is the book I would have been able to buy when we first got Eddie's diagnosis, that could have helped us through the early years of Eddie's life.

Although I appreciate that routines are not for everyone, and indeed some parents may feel that routines can make their children even more resistant to change, I really have found them invaluable for our family over the past two decades. I hope some, if not all, of them will help you as much as they have helped us.

However, it cannot be underestimated how difficult overcoming some of the issues can be, so try to ignore anyone who belittles your attempts or says you are making the situation more difficult than it is – as parents and carers, we know how difficult it is for our children and for us. I am sure these scenarios will ring true for many of you:

- 'Calm down and leave him alone – he will eat it eventually, when he is hungry enough!'

- 'Make him wait – how difficult can that be?' (Er, very difficult for an autistic person when they don't know what they are waiting for!)

- 'Why is that child rolling around on the floor? Tell him to get up.' (Well, if it was that easy, don't you think I would?)

When giving my talks, I always start with the well-known phrase, 'If you have met one autistic child then you have met one autistic child,' because it is so true. Despite the triad of impairments necessary for an ASD diagnosis, our children with autism are often very, very different to one another. For example:

- verbal/non-verbal

- can't talk/can't stop talking

- loves cuddles/can't bear to be touched

Therefore, how irritating is it when so many people ask me what Eddie's 'special powers' are? What's he a genius at? Aren't all autistic people savants, such as the character with an amazing memory depicted in *Rain Man*? I bet he is fantastic with numbers! Well, perhaps he does like numbers in the CBeebies programme *NumberJacks*, he totally understands the scoring system in snooker and has now learned his times tables, but he is not a maths genius: he can't speak clearly, has a communication disorder, huge sensory issues, behavioural issues and is a very vulnerable person, as he has very little understanding of the world around him; he will need round-the-clock care for his entire life!

Part 1

Routines for Everyday Life Skills

Introduction

What Is This Book About and Why Is It Different?

Children with autism and/or learning difficulties often need specific help to learn many of the life skills and behaviours that other children acquire naturally through everyday activities and interactions. Teaching these in a structured way, by breaking them down into component parts and reinforcing the routines with visual prompts and pictures, can really help. So this book includes numerous basic routines that are useful for home, and some for specific outings, to help prepare your child.

Every child is different so there is, of course, no guarantee that these routines will work in the same way for all children, but they do provide a place to start. When your child first gets a diagnosis, and you can see that they have a different way of learning, it is so important that you have a framework you can start with and some strategies to try, though you may need to adapt a given routine, or present it in a different way, to personalise it for your child.

This book aims to be useful in supporting carers and parents to establish doable and sustainable routines at home. In turn, this will help address various issues that parents who care for children with autism face and help the children to acquire strategies for daily living as well as valuable life skills. Establishing routines can also help to lessen your child's anxiety, as will be explained later in this introduction.

Many self-help books for parents of children with autism cover the issues that can be problematic. However, often a personalised routine is required to really help each individual child. That's where this book can help because it provides step-by-step, hands-on practical solutions. It includes many easy-to-follow sample routines that can be personalised for your child, as well as Social Stories™ that can also be adapted.

Who Might Find This Book Useful?

This book is aimed at anyone parenting or caring for children with autism and/or learning difficulties. Professionals, therapists and other practitioners will also find this resource useful in helping children they are working with, to complement and signpost support for the young people in their care.

In particular, this handbook is for parents and carers whose child has just received a diagnosis and who are looking for some practical help with difficulties they might be encountering, either at home or when out and about. Although it is impossible to generalise, as the approaches and solutions that work best for one child may not work for another, this book will give you a place to start, which will make it feel less daunting to try new routines and strategies that may help you and your child. This book shares my practical experience of real issues and instances from over the last 21 years, which will hopefully feel familiar to you as you work through it. It also aims to:

- put in context why your child may be finding things like washing and eating difficult

- give you some practical ideas that you can individualise for your child

- reassure you that, even if a strategy doesn't work the first time, it's OK to stand back and then try again.

How Is This Book Organised?

This book will describe and give clear examples of many of the most useful routines I have used to help Eddie acquire various everyday skills and to provide a framework/structure to his day. Many of the skills outlined are those needed for life at home, especially when getting ready in the morning and at bedtime, as well as eating and hygiene skills. The book also provides some routines for trips out, medical visits and a selection of unusual events, such as birthday parties, going to the beach, and so on.

Each routine includes a preparation section; preparation is important when starting to work with your child on implementing a new routine, and may well involve you testing out some ideas beforehand. There are tips to help problem-solve why a strategy may not be working, and there are also short sections on communication, visual support and self-care; these will in all likelihood be relevant to you as a parent of a child, or children, with autism, and will provide a starting point for gaining insight into these areas.

Throughout the book there are Eddie Story Boxes. These are anecdotes about events we have experienced with Eddie: some will be sad, some will be humorous, some will tell you how a particular skill was developed or how badly a routine or event went wrong. I hope these stories will help to bring this book to life and support you with your journey with your child – especially if things don't go to plan the first time.

Finally, there are some thoughts on you, the parent or carer, and any siblings in your family. The balance and complexity of family life is understandably different and more difficult with an autistic child. There are certainly plenty of positives, but it is also important to acknowledge the difficulties and ensure that siblings are given the time and attention they need too.

Why Routines Could be Helpful for Your Child

Establishing routines for children with autism can be really helpful: repeating the same routine for a particular activity reinforces the necessary behaviour, helps the learning process and, importantly, reduces anxiety of the unknown by giving the child confidence in and certainty about what is going to happen and when it will end. Routines may help with:

- learning new activities

- learning life skills

- going to new places

- transitioning from one activity to another

- coping with change.

Children with autism thrive on predictability and structure. But, as we know, the world is often chaotic, unpredictable and doesn't make sense to them, causing anxiety and meltdowns. So, by offering structure and routine throughout the day, and in various new or regular situations, the anxiety caused can be managed and lessened, hopefully making the day or the activity more enjoyable or, at the very least, more tolerable.

Also, establishing good routines helps make transitions, such as introducing a new carer or family member or change of school, more manageable, as the people involved can be advised of the routine and how to use it; such continuity makes the change of situation more seamless for both carer(s) and child. This will, in turn, give you confidence that your child will have a better experience and be able to cope with the change.

If no routines exist, each time you try to perform a daily sequence of events it might be carried out slightly differently; this can be confusing for your child, take longer and be more upsetting for everyone, leading to more frequent meltdowns.

It's worth saying that too much strict routine, and an expectation that things will always work out as planned, can become a problem if the person being cared for finds it impossible to deviate from a rigid set of activities, or move on to the next task if something they expected to happen hasn't occurred. It's a question of striking a balance: accommodate routines but, if possible, keep adding to or tweaking them so that deviation from the routine doesn't cause more anxiety and stress than you were trying to avoid in the first place. Therefore, purposefully sabotaging a routine and instilling a degree of flexibility and adaptability is useful, too, and will be referred to again later in Part 2. However, in my experience, the longer the routine has been in place the more relaxed Eddie is if one aspect changes.

Occasionally routines might not go to plan, as there will invariably be factors that are out of your control, plus it will take time for the routine to become established for you and your child. Don't get stressed or disheartened if it takes time, and always be prepared to tweak the plan if you find that it can work better when carried out slightly differently.

Eddie Story

As part of our shower and bedtime routine, I always laid out Eddie's pyjamas in the bathroom so he could get dressed after his shower. One day he arrived in the bathroom holding his pyjamas, which he had collected himself from his bedroom. I was so pleased he had done this for himself, and gave him lots of praise, and now he does this every time.

Each routine outlined in this book contains elements of others; for example, the 'Starting the Day' routine includes getting up, teeth cleaning, toileting and bag-packing schedules. These are clearly signposted, as you may want to learn the individual routines separately before adding them all together. Of course, if you already have an established routine for one of the elements then stick with that, if it works for you and your child.

The process of learning routines is not a one-off – keep doing them every day, if possible, completing the set of activities in the same sequence each time. Some routines may be learned and become embedded in your daily schedule very quickly, whereas others take more time. Once a routine is established, you may be able to withdraw the visual prompts, the sentence prompts (as a list) or you may need to keep them. You may also find you can expand the routine, or that your child expands it for you, by adding the step of putting dirty clothes in the laundry basket after a bath, for example.

Remember that, even once a routine has been learned and mastered, you may still need to direct/prompt the start of the routine, or a certain stage/stages of it, to keep your child on task. But ultimately, they may learn to follow it without your help.

The other point to bear in mind is that your child may have developed their own rituals for carrying out tasks, which they NEED to follow; you will need to be aware of these and allow time for them to be completed. Giving your child a countdown (5, 4, 3, 2, 1) can be very useful in warning your child or allowing them time to complete their own routine and rituals.

Finally, busy parents and carers have other commitments. Don't feel bad or get stressed if you can't perform a routine every day, or if some days things don't work out. That's life. Start again the next day, or soon after, so as not to undo all the good work you have already done.

Chapter 1

How to Implement a Routine

The sample routines in each section work for our family and for Eddie. It is not suggested that you copy these exactly; rather you can use the framework, format and ideas provided and adapt and personalise them for your child.

Planning

We quickly found that, to get Eddie to co-operate, we needed to make it very clear to him what he was working towards – if he didn't see the need or the point, it became increasingly difficult to engage him. For example, why would Eddie even think about what happens before food arrives on his plate? It's there, he eats it and that is that. Why would Eddie want to come on a walk? What is the point? He just doesn't understand why you would go on a walk as an experience on its own, or for its own enjoyment. The activity needs a beginning and an end, and, ideally, a purpose. In contrast, he totally understands a game of tenpin bowling: everyone has a turn, you knock down the skittles, you get 10 turns each, and then that is the end of the game. A beginning and a finite end – all very logical.

So we needed to break the activity down into stages, put it in context, step by step, for him to properly participate in the process and to make it more meaningful to him. A three-step approach has worked for us:

1. Goal Setting: What is the point? E.g. go to the dentist for a teeth inspection/ check-up

2. Clear Structure: What is the plan? E.g. pre-plan, routine, Social Story™

3. Incentive: What is the reward? E.g. activity, food treat, special toy

Of course, with some of the hygiene routines, your child may simply want to get them out of the way as quickly as possible so they can get on to the next or preferred activity. However, finishing a task and moving on to the favoured activity will be reinforcing in itself. (Reinforcers are explained in more detail below.)

This planning stage is really important because it can help you to think through the whole process, plan what you need and be prepared. Choosing a meaningful reinforcer/incentive is key too.

The incentive will obviously vary for each child but will usually involve the offer of a favourite sensory toy, fidget toy, a favourite activity or similar, because, generally, children with ASD are not motivated simply by social feedback from others. Therefore, you may want to have specific reinforcers that you keep just for routines, so that they remain desirable to your child.

We found it was best to avoid too many food-based incentives because, quite often, a particular food becomes associated too strongly with the completion of the routine, and this might cause a problem if that food is not available. However, if snacks generally work for your child, go with them.

Presentation

You need to decide how you will present the stages of the routine to your child. Because children with autism are often visual learners, using pictures that are uncluttered and easy to understand will work well. You can then use the same visuals for timetables, choice boards and to depict the stages of a routine. Some visuals also include the written word under the picture to help children to read the word as well as understand the picture.

What visuals will you use to reinforce the routine? Ideally, you would use the same type of visuals that you use for any other visual prompt work that you might be doing with your child, to help with continuity. These could be symbols that you have purchased or downloaded, photos, or whatever your child will prefer. See Pictorial and Visual Support in Chapter 4 for more information about using visuals.

Make the routine into a Social Story™ if you are already using Social Stories™ and finding them effective for your child. (There is more information about Social Stories™ in Chapter 3.) Another idea is to present words in a list, heading by heading, with brief instructions of what will happen. Again, how you present the routine will depend on what works best for your child.

Timing

At What Age?

Deciding when to start the routine is important: you may wish to do it when a situation or activity has already become very difficult, to stop the problem escalating and the associated behaviour becoming embedded.

Eddie took to going to bed fairly easily but found going to the hairdresser very difficult indeed. We would have Eddie in his buggy, placed in the shop window so he could watch the buses and taxis go by, while the hairdresser manically tried to cut his hair, with every passer-by gazing in to watch the floor show – it was then that I realised we needed to try a different method.

Time Frame for Implementation

This needs to be considered because, depending on the routine you are trying to establish, it may take several months rather than days or weeks.

For example, a trip to the hairdresser happens every 6 to 8 weeks; therefore, you will only have the opportunity to practise and establish the routine every 6 to 8 weeks. On the other hand, the bedtime and morning routines happen every day and, while it might be a daily task to establish and tweak the routine, there will also be plenty of opportunity to do so.

Reflection and Progress Check

I can't emphasise strongly enough how important this stage of the process is. For some children, you may be trying to overcome many different issues that are coming into play: maybe sensory, maybe behavioural, stress and anxiety, or ability to understand. All of these combined can make implementing a routine very difficult for everyone involved, as well as imposing a new structure or set of rules to cope with, even if, in the longer term, it will make your child's life easier or more tolerable.

All of the preparation, planning and visuals described above, will help to ease the transition to the new routine; however, it may well be that something happens along the way and you need to stop to prioritise that issue, even if it means taking some time out from the routine. This obstacle could be related to practical, personal or family issues, or linked to a meltdown, for example. It is, of course, fine to take a break and then come back to a routine, but try not to leave it for too long, or you may have to start from the beginning again.

Eddie Story

Eddie has always been resistant to wearing clothes; as a toddler, he used to love to run around with no pants on. Once we got him to wear pants, it was then a struggle for him to wear long trousers. He still can't wear jumpers, or any item of clothing unless every label is cut out. Socks are also too restrictive and, ideally, he would go to school without them – even in his school shoes. Summer is better, in T-shirts and shorts. His default is to wear pyjamas all day, to indicate that he has no intention of leaving the house!

We do have Undressing and Dressing routines – complete with 'dirty washing in the laundry basket', 'clean clothes in his drawers', 'pyjamas on the bed, ready for bedtime' – but every now and then, at weekends and during holidays, we let it go, just to let Eddie make his own decision and, as a treat, wear his pyjamas all day in the house.

Chapter 2

Obstacles You May Encounter, and Solutions

Your child may have established their own routines, in their head, unbeknown to you; while you are giving verbal or even visual commands in the background, they may be focusing on completing their ritual or routine and are, therefore, not able to process what you are asking them to do. This may involve, for example, their own countdown or arranging toys or objects in a certain way; they will need to complete this activity before they can focus on the next task.

Scripting and stimming have been, and I think will continue to be, issues for Eddie and barriers to learning and engaging.

Stimming

'Stimming' is short for 'self-stimulation' and includes any number of repetitive behaviours, such as hand-flapping, jumping and fiddling. Many people stim but, with autistic children, the stimming can get in the way of their learning and their ability to complete everyday functions. However, rather than trying to stop them stimming, it is best to try to understand when and why your child needs it and what triggers this behaviour.

Stimming behaviours can block out things in the environment that are causing sensory overload in some way. They can also be helpful in providing sensory input when a person feels understimulated, as the repetitive behaviour provides the sensory feedback they need.

Stimming can indicate both negative and positive emotions, such as fear and anxiety or joy and excitement. So the behaviour should not always be considered negative, as it can aid self-regulation and expression. Unfortunately, as you will probably all be aware, these stimming behaviours are often seen by outsiders as 'weird', and sometimes people react by pointing or commenting; at school and other social venues, the behaviours can be viewed as disruptive. Clearly, if stimming behaviours involve head-banging, biting or other forms of self-harm, these need to be addressed.

Eddie Story

Eddie often sits with his fingers pressed into his ears and makes gurgling noises. People unfamiliar with him may mistakenly think he is blocking out noise, but I believe this stimming behaviour allows him to hear his gurgling noises, and that the vibration they make in his ears is comforting to him. This behaviour can indicate that he is experiencing joy and delight at something, but also that he is upset or angry. It can even be part of the process of him working up to do something he is scared of, for example, having a vaccination or bodily examination.

Scripting

Scripting is also a regulating behaviour that involves repetition, over and over again, of the same words or phrases. It is also known as 'echolalia': the person is merely echoing someone else's words, rather than speaking their own thoughts. The words can often be taken from conversations overheard, favourite programmes, films and books, or anything that is of particular interest or appeal.

While scripting is very satisfying and comforting for the person doing it, their attention is likely being completely taken away from the task in hand. This can limit learning and skill development, as the person's attention tends to be focused on the words they are saying, or the scene being remembered or played out in their head. They may need to be gently but firmly brought back to the instruction they are supposed to be listening to. Not only can scripting be a coping mechanism for when the person is anxious, confused or just not understanding what is required of them, but it can also be part of a routine that they are attaching to the activity you are asking them to perform.

Eddie Story

Eddie seems to have a whole library of scenes in his memory, which he recalls and plays out in his head when he is not looking at his screen. We are aware of this because he is concentrating very hard but not looking at us, as he visualises the scene running in his mind. He can be giggling away (and, again, someone not familiar with him may assume he is finding something in the room amusing, but he isn't; it's the scene in his head that is making him laugh). It is pointless carrying on at this point. If the situation is not time-critical we can let him finish scripting. If we need to get his attention straight away because, for instance, we are trying to leave the house, then we gently bring him back to the moment, getting direct eye contact and giving him a clear instruction such as 'Shoes on Eddie'; this ensures we have his full attention.

Stimming can be helped by monitoring the environment around your child for sensory triggers. For instance, whenever clapping or singing happens, Eddie will instantly want to stim to block it out. If he starts to stim or script, we try to continue to communicate and bring his focus back to what we are trying to do. Also, if he has done some really good work, concentrated for a reasonable period of time and completed his task, allowing him to stim following lots of praise can actually be a positive reward.

I remember very fondly, when Eddie was 6 years old, the head of the special school he was attending said to me, 'Lesley, it's perfectly fine to let him just be autistic for some of the time'. I think that was great advice.

This is a very basic introduction to stimming and scripting, and it is recommended that you seek professional advice if your child's stimming is really problematic and/ or harmful.

Sensory Issues and Triggers

The skills we are looking at teaching in this book often take place in an environment that is challenging from a sensory perspective and will need to be modified to provide the best opportunity for a positive outcome. For example, there will be bright lights, the noise of running water, and strong smells in the bathroom and kitchen, strong smells and noises in the hairdressing salon, and so on.

Many people with autism have sensory issues which can overwhelm their ability to tolerate certain things, such as itchy clothes, loud noises, tastes and textures of food, smells, bright lights and crowded places. These can, if bad enough, trigger a meltdown, so this is why we need to factor them into any new routines. These issues will be highlighted in the sample routines, but the list is not exhaustive, so do add any possible sensory difficulties in the preparation phase.

As well as environmental factors, children with autism may be 'tactile defensive'. This means they have an increased sensitivity to touch – either to them touching things or to things touching them. When this happens, they respond by pulling away or resisting any contact completely. Eddie has an aversion to plunging his hands into a basin of water to wash them: his hands and fingers tense and I need to lower them into the water gently, as they form a crab-like shape – however, he could spend all day jumping into a swimming pool!

Conversely, some children with autism may be 'sensory seekers', in that they might need more sensory input from their environment and, therefore, like jumping, flapping hands, spinning things or, in Eddie's case, chewing on things that are not meant to be eaten, such as sticky tack or the glue that attaches a straw to his carton of drink.

Eddie Story

When Eddie becomes overwhelmed, his reaction has always been to throw himself on the floor and kick his legs, like a ladybird that can't turn itself the right way up. This was manageable when he was little but, as he has grown older, it has become more difficult. It is also distressing, as it means he has reached a point at which he can't tolerate something and is very upset. We, therefore, need to try to anticipate and avoid scenarios which will cause him this reaction.

Weighted Therapy Products

Many children with ASD have sensory processing issues and can benefit from weighted therapy products; the extra pressure they provide can instil a sense of calm, rather like having a deep pressure massage on the shoulders or back that may relax your child or help ground them. Products range from a weighted jacket or blanket to a lap pad to be used in a classroom.

As with all strategies, weighted products may not work for all children, but they are definitely worth trying because some people report the results as lifechanging; for example, using a weighted blanket may have helped a child, who used to have great difficulty sleeping, to sleep through the night.

A weighted blanket can also be used to wrap around a distressed child to help calm them and make them feel safe. Weighted jackets can be worn to give a child the constant feeling of pressure to help relax them and help them to concentrate better.

Alternatively, think about whether your child likes wearing a backpack. Try it out by getting them to wear one with bottles of water or books inside to make it a bit heavier. This is a quick and easy way of trying weighted therapy. If your child is calmed by this, then other forms of weighted therapy may also work for them.

Sensory Direct UK offer a hire scheme for weighted blankets, so you can trial a blanket with your child, to see if it works, before you decide to buy; this is helpful as they tend to be quite expensive. You can also buy them VAT-free, if purchased for a disabled child.

Ideally, you should consult an occupational therapist for an assessment to determine whether your child has sensory processing issues and if they could benefit from weighted therapy.

Chapter 3

Techniques to Support Routines

Timers

Time is a particularly abstract concept for children, and especially for children with autism, so using visual timers at home and school is an ideal way of making the concept of time more accessible. As the timer counts down, this helps to represent the passing of time in a concrete and visual way, which makes it easier to understand and work with.

There are various types of timers that can be used for behaviour management and to help with routines. Sand timers are the most popular, but there are other visual or digital timers that some children prefer as they get older.

Using timers can be another way of reducing uncertainty in your child's day, by adding another brick to the framework that keeps them feeling safe and less anxious.

Sand Timers

Sand timers are ideal for helping children to develop an understanding of time and can support with routines, too.

Sand timers work because they:

- help with understanding the concept of time
- offer a visual representation of the amount of time elapsed
- offer a visual representation of the amount of time left
- can help a child to wait
- can help a child accept that an activity has to finish
- can be used to practise turn-taking.

Many sand timers are colour-coded, so your child can learn to recognise the colour and associate it with a particular length of time: green is one minute, yellow is three minutes, blue is five minutes, and so on.

Younger children will need shorter timers to begin with (1, 2, 3 and 5 minutes) – 5 minutes is actually a long time for a child to wait, concentrate or understand. Select a timer for the longest possible time you think your child can tolerate. Try introducing one timer at a time so they get used to the length of time.

So, perhaps, a 1-minute timer could be used for waiting for something to happen – such as getting in the bath, getting out of the bath, cleaning teeth, or lights out at bedtime. The 3-minute timer could be used to countdown that an activity has to finish or that you need to leave somewhere. Or, perhaps, if you have trouble getting your child out of bed in the morning, the yellow 3-minute timer could be used to indicate three more minutes of lie-in before they need to get up.

Sand timers representing longer times of 10, 15 and 30 minutes may be useful for situations such as taking turns on devices, getting a child to practise a musical instrument, doing homework or completing a meal.

Other Types of Timers

Digital timers – these types of timers show time numerically, and can be set to either count up or down and then sound a bleeping alarm once the set time has been reached. Digital timers tend to be small and portable.

Time Timer® – this brightly coloured, numbered timer shows time elapsing visually; as time passes, the coloured disc becomes smaller to show how much time is left.

Time Tracker® – this device has colour-coded lights – red, yellow and green – rather like a set of traffic lights, which give a visual indication of how much time is left.

Clocks

As well as understanding timing devices, such as those detailed above, it is a useful skill if your child can tell the time using either a clock face or a digital 24-hour clock. This will further allow you to help structure their day and give certainty about when activities will be happening, which, again, helps to reassure them and reduce anxiety.

Visual Timetables

Quite often children with autism are visual learners and, if their receptive language is delayed or disordered, it can really help to have clear, uncluttered and familiar pictures, photos or symbols to underpin what it is you are telling them or asking them to do.

Very early on, we found that it helped enormously to give Eddie as many details as possible about what would be happening in the future. In the same way, a timetable is usually provided at school, such visual timetables can be used at home for daily activities, both during the week and at the weekend, using pictures or symbols or photographs – or a mixture of all three – depending on the child's level of understanding. For consistency, it would be useful to find out what visual support system your child's nursery or school are using with them.

- Make sure the visuals are large enough for your child to see and understand; don't compromise on the size of the planner or timetable – make it large enough so it can accommodate the size of visuals your child needs. Our first visual timetable was the side of a huge cardboard box.

- Keep the timetable somewhere accessible so it can be seen and referred to.

- Personalise the planner with a picture of your child and some stickers, etc.

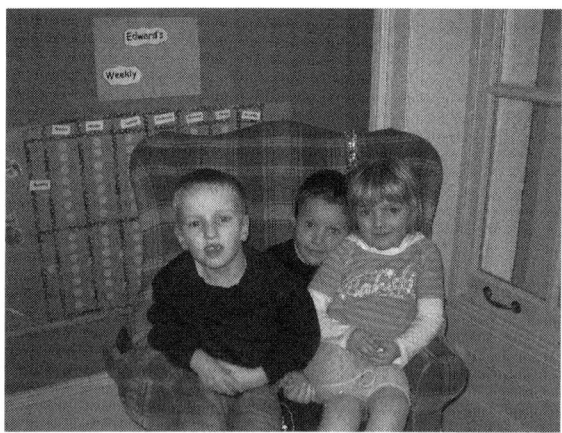

Eddie with his visual timetable

Visual Timetables are particularly effective because they are simple to follow, visual not wordy and allow flexibility, as they can be amended if a plan changes.

Something we found quite useful was that, if Eddie didn't like the activity, he would pull off the activity card; this gave us an indication, or warning, that he didn't want to do it or that it involved something that was potentially going to be a problem.

As your child progresses and starts to be able to read, they may not need visuals on their timetable but can have the schedule for the day listed with a time or clock face by each activity.

There are also various digital planners and apps that can be loaded onto smartphones and iPads to provide structure and routine. These may or may not be the way you want to go with your young child, especially if it's likely to cause confusion between the device they play on and the device you are using for managing routines and visual schedules. You will know best what will work for your child.

A Diary

We have found that it has helped enormously to give as much detail as possible to Eddie about what will be happening in the future. Initially, this was on a daily basis but, as he got older, we found that having his own diary, containing key dates and events, really helped to prepare him and manage his expectations. We just used a plain A5 diary and helped him to print off lots of pictures of things to stick on the front of it to personalise it. He chose snooker balls, Pingu, chocolate, tenpin bowling and a picture of himself! Key dates to include:

- school/college terms

- holidays, if we are going away

- short breaks

- his birthday and all family members' birthdays

- any treatments, or dental appointments

- haircuts

- school trips

- sessions with a support worker

We also use the diary to show if a different member of the family will be getting him up or putting him to bed on certain days, so that he won't be surprised or made anxious by the change to his usual routine.

As he has got older, we have encouraged him to write the entries in himself, and it is quite revealing because he will cross out an entry that he is not looking forward to or doesn't want to do. This is a helpful pointer to us that some additional preparation for that day will be necessary.

The diary was particularly important during the Coronavirus lockdowns of 2020 and 2021, as Eddie would be continually referring to it to see if events had been crossed out or added. Of course, it was really difficult, because we could give him no certainty: we had no idea when schools would be opening or when any of the activities he enjoys, such as swimming, going to the gym, crazy golf, seeing his support worker, could be resumed. By Easter, a month into lockdown, the only thing I could actually say would be happening for certain, was his birthday in August.

Having the diary then became a good tool for communication and interaction, as we would look through the pages and talk about the activities, and I would try to reassure Eddie that things would be OK, even if these activities weren't going to happen.

Social Stories™

Social Stories™ were originally developed in the USA by Carol Gray and they are used to help children with autism to understand new or challenging social situations. We have used these extensively with Eddie: they have made a real difference to what he can and can't tolerate and help to manage his expectations of what will happen, especially if we are doing something or going somewhere for the first time.

Details of where to find more information about Social Stories™ are included at the back of this book, but there are a variety of resources, from books such as *My Social Stories Book* by Carol Gray and Abbie Leigh White (2002, Jessica Kingsley Publishers), to software that enables you to write a Social Story™ and will also produce the pictures to go with it. You will be writing the story for your child, whom you know best; therefore, once you can see the format, structure and the language to use, you should have the confidence to write one yourself.

Your child's school or nursery may also be able to produce them for you with the graphics, if they have the software, as many schools now use Social Stories™. Here are some tips for writing your own Social Stories™:

- What is the purpose of the story and why do you need it?

- Aim to use succinct, short sentences and no 'flowery' language.

- Personalise the story for your child by using their name.

- Identify and refer to the things your child might be wary of or anxious about.

- Use very reassuring language to reinforce that your child will be OK.

- Do your research if visiting somewhere new, so you can refer, for example, to the layout of a room or the colour of a door to make it familiar.

- Give an indication of how long the event or activity might take.

- Acknowledge any emotions your child might be feeling.

- Use pictures, photos or symbols if your child cannot read or benefits from pictorial support.

The sample Social Story™ below is for a young person who is not keen on wearing appropriate clothes for the seasons, and, in this example, they are encouraged to wear a jumper when it gets cold.

1. Read through the Social Story™ with your child, with the jumper or sweatshirt you want them to wear to school or wherever it is they are going.

2. Go through the Social Story™ several times; show you will be pleased if your child wears the jumper.

3. When your child has managed to achieve the goal of the Social Story™, use that experience to remind them that what is stated as happening in the Social Story™ will actually happen and that when you use Social Stories™ they will be OK. They will then learn that Social Stories™ are a strategy that can be relied upon.

Sample Social Story™ for Putting on Another Layer of Clothing (e.g. a Jumper)

- It is very cold in winter.
- Sometimes we need to wear a jumper or a sweatshirt.
- Wearing a jumper is OK.
- I will feel warm if I wear a jumper.
- I want to feel warm. I don't want to feel cold.
- I can choose a jumper I like.
- Wearing a jumper is OK.
- I can wear a jumper on the bus.
- I can wear a jumper at school.
- I will be OK wearing my jumper.
- When I get home, I can take my jumper off.
- But I must wear my jumper when I am out of the house.
- I might get very cold and become ill if I don't wear my jumper.
- I don't want to be ill.
- So I will wear my jumper.
- I will be OK wearing my jumper.
- My jumper will keep me warm.

The example hopefully illustrates the format and language to use, depending on the needs of your child, the subject and situation.

This Social Story™ can, of course, apply to any item of clothing, such as socks, outer coat or gloves. Once you have established the format, you can re-use it to cater for a different scenario.

A Social Story™ will be provided for each routine that we feature in this book.

Social Stories™ have been, and continue to be, an amazing tool to support Eddie both at home and at school. They can be used for literally any situation, whether it's explaining the fact that the school bus that is coming next week will be blue rather than green, to explaining why face masks and sanitising were required due to Covid-19. It's a tried and tested framework that is in common usage in the autism world, thankfully.

Verbal Countdown, Tick Lists and Reward Systems

There are various tried and tested strategies I refer to throughout the book, which we have picked up from nursery, school and therapists. Not all of them will work for everyone but they may give you further ideas for supporting your child.

Verbal Countdown

I have mentioned sand timers as a countdown tool to show that an activity must finish. In addition, or if you aren't using/don't have access to a timer (if, for example, you are out and about) then a verbal countdown (5, 4, 3, 2, 1) can be very effective.

Countdowns are commonly used in classrooms, when the teacher wants everyone to be quiet so the lesson can start, but they can also be helpful for our children because people with autism quite often have difficulty with transitioning from one activity to another. If they are very focused on what they are doing, then using lots of words, such as 'Come in quickly, we are going to be late' or 'Come on, I have told you three times now, we need to go', can be overwhelming for them, as this is a lot of language to process. A simple countdown – 5, 4, 3, 2, 1 – in a firm voice, if used frequently to indicate that it's time to move on to the next activity, can result in timely compliance by your child.

Tick Lists

Several of the routines require a number of things to be picked up, packed or remembered, and these lists can clutter up the visual timetable if they appear there. Therefore, it can be helpful to have a separate check list, or tick list, that your child can refer to, ticking off each item when they have dealt with it. Here are some examples:

School bag

☐ lunchbox

☐ drinks bottle

☐ iPad/AAC device/iPod

☐ charger

☐ home to school book

☐ homework holder

☐ fidget item/comforter/favourite book or toy

☐ chewy tube

☐ wallet/purse with bus pass

☐ ID on lanyard, if appropriate

☐ ear defenders

Packed lunch

☐ sandwich

☐ rice cake

☐ banana

☐ yoghurt

☐ grapes

☐ Milky Way

☐ juice carton

PE bag

☐ training shoes

☐ football boots

☐ shorts

☐ shirt

☐ socks

☐ wash bag

☐ towel

Wash bag

☐ shampoo

☐ deodorant

☐ body spray

☐ flannel/sponge

Chapter 3

Print or write out the list and laminate it, or write it on a wipe-clean board, so you can re-use it many times by just erasing the ticks.

Tick lists can be helpful as they:

- serve as a reminder to your child
- may lessen the number of times items are forgotten or lost
- help your child to be more self-sufficient
- speed up the getting-ready-to-leave process.

Reward Systems

How you reward your child is a hugely personal thing because it depends so much on what will actually:

- motivate them at the outset
- encourage them to keep going
- make them feel satisfied they have been adequately rewarded once they have completed the task or mastered the routine
- make them feel proud of what they have achieved.

The rewards should also be appropriate for and accessible to your particular child, and reflect the significance of what your child is being asked to achieve. Reward charts where children receive a sticker/star to reinforce good behaviour, for example, each time they complete a task or try extra hard, can be very powerful for some children but too abstract and meaningless for others. Extra computer time or time on a device is very tangible and can be motivating for some; being given the choice of a new sensory toy from the goody box might be more persuasive for others.

Eddie often expects to receive a sticker from a health professional – it's almost part of his routine to not leave the room until he has been offered a sticker, chosen a sticker and stuck it on himself. For major one-off achievements, like having a vaccination, chocolate buttons would be the reward I use.

Chapter 4
Why Is Communication Important for a Routine?

Speaking and Communicating

To diagnose a person as having autism they must present with the triad of impairments. Namely difficulties with:

- social interaction

- social communication

- restrictive and repetitive patterns of behaviour.

Some, but not all, autistic people are unable to speak, such as Eddie was, or have very limited speech. Others can repeat what other people say but do not actually understand what it means; this is called echolalia.

I think it is totally understandable for parents to become very focused on a child's lack of speech. Not least because it's a developmental milestone in young children and a vitally important life skill, but also because you want to be able to converse with your child.

However, once it becomes clear that speech is not going to come quickly, due to a speech delay or disorder, there are other things you can do to communicate with your child.

Eddie Story

A very wise speech therapist taught me exactly this. I was getting very frustrated with Eddie and kept mouthing, 'Say "Mum," Eddie, say "Mum Mum Mum Mmmum,"' and, of course, he ignored me and looked away at something else – as though he was deaf and had not heard me. The therapist pointed out that it takes many, many connections in the brain, as well as the muscles in the mouth and the tongue, for speech to be possible and, in Eddie's case, these pathways were not quite developed yet. But she also told me there were lots of other things we could focus on, because actual word sounds are the final building block towards speech, not the first.

The Communication Pyramid graphic below illustrates how communication develops and shows simply, from the bottom up, how speech and language are supported by other skills. The foundation of communication is good attention and listening skills.

Communication Pyramid

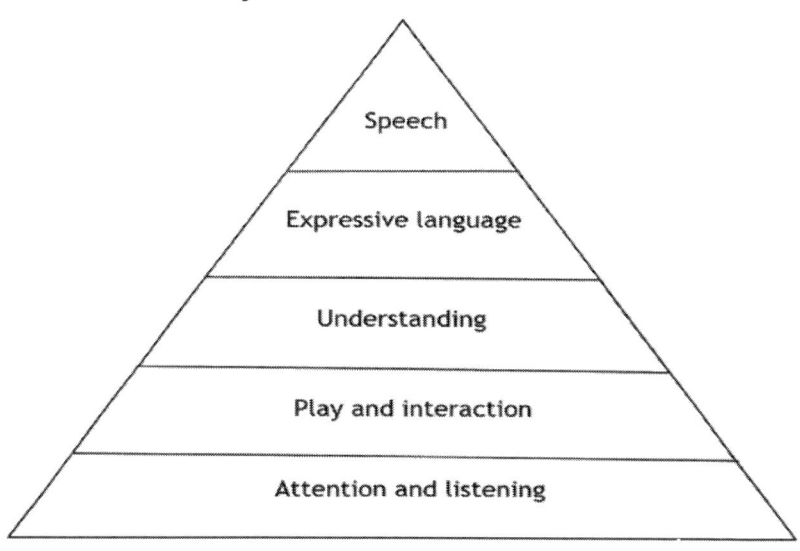

Speech

Expressive language

Understanding

Play and interaction

Attention and listening

Good eye contact is needed to help your child focus on what you are doing or saying: this is also where visual prompts can be used to help support what it is you are talking about or instructing them to do.

Eddie had single-channelled attention control for activities that he enjoyed. So when he was focused on an activity, be it a very repetitive one, such as lining up cars or balls, both his visual and auditory channels were involved, and he would resist or ignore any gentle attempt to try and direct his play or interrupt what he was doing.

Therefore, to play and interact with him we needed to get his full attention, and the best way to do that was to be doing or holding something that he was interested in.

We tried all the classic eye contact techniques, such as peek-a-boo, blowing bubbles, letting go of blown-up balloons, cause-and-effect toys and countdowns, to help build up his ability to make eye contact and focus. The idea behind these techniques being that you don't let go of the balloon or blow the bubbles or let the ball run down the ramp until your child has looked at you.

All these strategies can be fun and engaging, and led to us trying to teach Eddie a non-verbal, visual-based form of communication (PECS) while we waited to see if speech would develop over time.

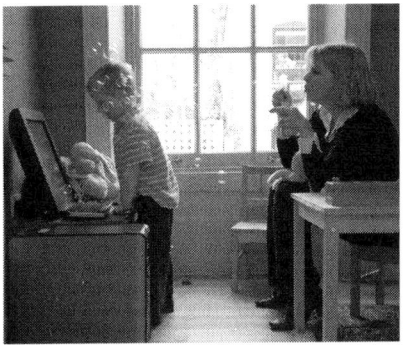 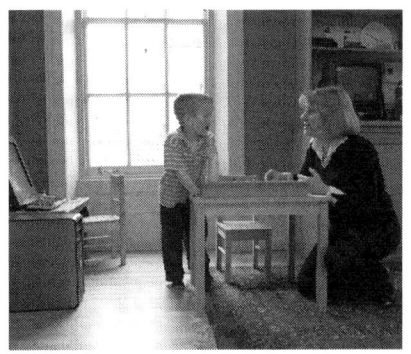

How NOT to do table top work and Eddie enjoying table top work

Non-verbal Language Support

We got an informal diagnosis – that Eddie was likely to have a communication disorder, rather than being deaf – when he was 18 months old. Then we were given the following advice:

- Seek a formal diagnosis from the Child Development Team.

- Early intervention is imperative – seek a place at a special needs nursery/ school.

- Start using the Picture Exchange Communication System (PECS).

- Learn Makaton sign language.

Many people refer to picture symbols and timetable symbols – in fact, any picture symbols – as using PECS, but this is not correct. PECS is a process that MUST involve the giving of a card in exchange for a requested item; it's a two-way process, requiring two people, as explained below.

The Picture Exchange Communication System (PECS)

Phase 1: How to communicate
A person learns to hand over a single picture to another person and then receive an item or activity they really want from that person.

E.g. Child gives a picture of a cracker to his mother who gives him a cracker probably while sitting opposite each other at a table.

Phase 2: Distance and persistence

A person learns to generalise this skill by moving to pick up the picture and then moving to the other person to hand it over and receive the item requested.

E.g. Child moves to pick up the cracker symbol from the table and takes it to his mother who is sitting on the sofa holding the cracker.

Phase 3: Picture discrimination

A person learns to choose from two or more pictures to ask for desired items.

E.g. Child picks a picture from a choice board that may have several pictures of food items or toys he particularly likes.

Phase 4: Sentence structure

The 'I want' card is introduced and a person learns to use this card plus a picture card to make a simple sentence.

E.g. The 'I want' card is added to the choice board, and the child picks up that card plus the picture of the cracker and takes it to his mother who is holding a cracker, and she hands over the cracker.

Phase 5: Responsive requesting

A person learns to use PECS to answer questions, such as 'What do you want?', and the communication becomes a 3 stage process. Mother, then child, then mother.

E.g. Mother asks child 'What do you want?' and child picks up the 'I want' card and the cracker card picture card to request the item. Mother gives him the cracker.

Phase 6: Commenting

A person learns to comment in response to questions, other than 'What do you want?'

These might include 'What can you see?', 'What can you hear?'

This is quite a step up, as it doesn't involve an exchange of an item and is not underpinned by fulfilling a request.

What is required to trial PECS?
What you will need:

- two adults
- a table

- a picture symbol of an item your child really likes/desires
- the item depicted on the picture symbol

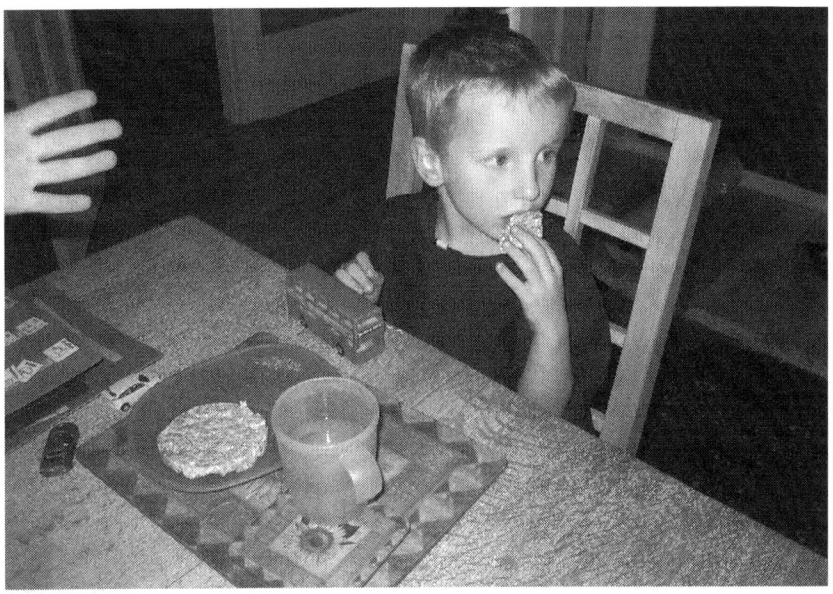

Eddie using PECS at mealtime

For Eddie, we chose his favourite snack – Thai Bite Crackers – for the item he would request, each cracker broken into three pieces, as we would repeat the exchange many times and probably consume a whole packet of crackers during this session.

What you will do:

To start, sit one adult at one side of the table, with your child and the other adult on the opposite side of the table.

The adult on the opposite side of the child holds a piece of cracker.

The picture card with the symbol is placed in front of the child.

The adults model 'the exchange' by helping the child to pick up the card and give it to the adult holding the cracker.

The adult says, 'cracker', and hands the child the cracker. The child eats it.

On receiving the card, the adult must hand over the cracker immediately, as a quick response validates the request and makes it meaningful.

Repeat this process, but on the third occasion wait for the child to pick up the picture card to give it to the adult holding out the cracker.

27

Eddie Story

Eddie was actually very young to be starting to use PECS, but we were keen to try it out as soon as possible.

Eddie took to it immediately and we must have completed about 50 exchanges with bits of cracker and about 30 with chocolate buttons in the first session alone. I think this may have been, not just because of the items we chose, but also because it played to Eddie's liking of repetition!

In terms of communication, this was a huge breakthrough for us because it showed that Eddie:

- had the cognitive ability to learn
- had the desire to communicate if the item was appealing enough
- could remember the steps required for the exchange.

We soon started using other picture symbols to request items, anything tangible that could be handed over in exchange for the correct picture symbol: mostly favourite food items and favourite toys. We then extended this to having two or three picture cards in front of him, so that he was required to decide which item he wanted to request.

An additional benefit we found with PECS was that, as the item was being handed over, Eddie would make eye contact with us: that, too, was a huge step forward as, like many children with autism, he would usually avoid eye contact. By having eye contact with him at the point of the handover, the exchange became a social interaction as well as a communicative one.

Within a year, we were able to move on to the persistence and distance phase and 6 months later to making a choice between two and then three picture cards in front of him. Making him move to find the person to hand over the picture further reinforced his desire to obtain what he wanted. Giving him a choice of two then three cards to decide which item to request made him focus just that little bit longer on the cards to discriminate the pictures.

I believe that all of these skills, practised daily through PECS, transformed Eddie's ability and desire to communicate in his formative years – a really positive example of early intervention.

For PECS to be effective

For PECS to be effective, you need to be absolutely rigorous and methodical.

- An exchange of picture for item must take place.

- Only the item that matches the picture symbol card offered can be handed over. For example, if there are two cards in front of your child and they hand you the cracker card but reach for the banana, you must hand them the cracker and say 'cracker'.

The beauty of PECS is that it starts at the most basic level – one picture card to request one item – and builds up to communicate whole sentences. Also, there can be no confusion about what is being requested because the picture shows what is being asked for.

Once Eddie had shown an ability to use PECS, we were able to start using other forms of visual prompts and visual timetables. And again, the advantage of visual communication is that it is less confusing because the picture shows exactly what is being requested or which activity will be happening. This can help to give certainty and reduce anxiety in a world that is often very confusing and worrying for our children.

More information on PECS can be obtained from www.pecs-unitedkingdom.com

Pictorial and Visual Support

As shown throughout this book, visuals can be a crucial aid for kick-starting and improving communication skills.

In addition, providing pictures to support instructions, routines and timetables can be invaluable for increasing understanding and lessening anxiety about what is going to happen.

Visual Timetable

A visual timetable is a chart that uses pictures, symbols and/or photographs, attached by hook-and-loop fasteners (such as Velcro®), to show the activities that will be happening that day, and in what order. Initially, it does not need to show the time the activity will happen, as it is literally the sequence in which the events will occur that needs to be reinforced to your child. The beauty of a visual timetable is that your child can keep looking at it for reassurance and to check that they have understood.

The timetable can be set up either for the whole day or, more usually for younger children, it can be broken down to show just the morning activities, then set up for the afternoon activities and, finally, for the evening schedule.

Chapter 4

For children who need greater support, you can have a separate 'Now and Next Board'. Using the same symbols that you are using every day in your visual timetable, you show what activity your child is doing now and what activity they will be doing next. It is a simple way of breaking down the timetable into a shorter form, to help your child focus on the task they are currently doing. For example:

NOW	NEXT
Have a Bath	Clean Teeth
Clean Teeth	Go to Park
Dinner	Play on Computer

Types of Visuals

There are a variety of symbols or pictures that can be purchased, and a quick internet search will bring up suggestions of how to make your own or where to buy readymade systems. In addition to the visuals for the activity timetable, there are also various pictorial aids that can be bought for the routines you will be implementing.

A choice, then, has to be made as to whether you are going to use pictures, photographs or symbols, and this will depend on which medium your child responds to best. For consistency, it would be useful to find out what visual support system the nursery or school are using with your child.

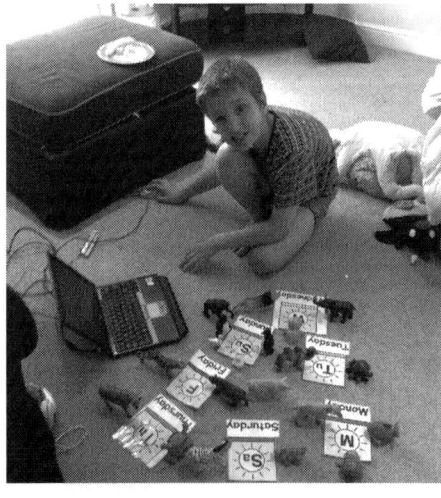

Playing a game

Part 2
Sample Strategies and Routines

Introduction to Sample Routines

Establishing routines for children with autism can be very helpful: repeating the same routine for a particular activity reinforces the behaviour necessary for that task, it helps the learning process and, importantly, it reduces anxiety of the unknown because following the same routine gives the child confidence in and certainty of what is going to happen and when it will end.

The situations we will cover in this book are as follows:

- Home to school
- Packing a school bag
- Getting dressed
- Toileting
- Going out in the car
- Going to the hairdresser
- Going shopping
- Going to buy a pair of shoes
- Going for a walk
- Introducing new foods
- Mealtimes
- Eating out
- Helping out at home
- Going to the doctor
- Going to the dentist
- Going to the hospital (for an X-ray)
- Going for a vaccination
- Having a birthday party
- Going to the beach

- Having a photograph taken for a passport

- Going to an airport

- Bathtime/showering

- Brushing teeth

- Sleeping and bedtime

- Staying away from home overnight

These strategies are most appropriate for children aged from 2 to 11 years old, as they cover the early-years skills and situations you are likely to be encountering for the first time. There are some routines that may still be relevant for teenagers who, for a variety of reasons, have not mastered every stage of a particular routine or daily living skill.

Chapter 5
Starting the Day

Home to School

The weekday morning routine can be the most difficult, especially if you have more than one child. It is time critical, as you probably need to get to the childminder, nursery or school for a certain time. It also takes place early in the morning, when people may feel especially tired and sleepy, particularly after an unsettled night. But it's one of the most important routines to get right, as it sets everyone up for the day ahead – a bad start can set the tone for the rest of the day. So we try and aim for a calm and consistent routine, and, importantly, one that is achievable!

Our family has always benefitted from having a strict routine in the morning, as this seems to ensure Eddie has a good start to the day. This is helped by the fact that he has to go to school on Local Authority transport: the bus comes at the same time every day and that is what our routine is based around.

Planning

- The routine needs to be achievable, so allow enough time to complete the tasks and achieve the target departure time.

- Get up earlier than you wake your child, so you can do the packed lunch, etc. in a calm way, and not while you are trying to give your child breakfast!

- If you are working through a visual schedule or a tick list, show it to your child when they first wake up and refer to it as you work through the sequence of tasks.

- You may know or pre-empt the tasks that your child will find most difficult and need most support with: allow extra time for these and a bit of leeway, so that if things don't go to plan there is time to deal with it.

- If you have other children, let them know what the plan is so they can really help by co-operating and even assisting you.

- If third-party transport is involved, be sure to liaise with the driver and/or escort to ensure that you are made aware of any changes – see the Eddie Story Box on page 39.

Sample Routines

I have included a number of sample routines throughout the book, covering everything from helping your child to get ready in the morning to preparing them for bed in the evening. Each one, based on years of experience, stems from an individualised routine that has worked successfully with Eddie. I do hope that you will find it relatively easy to personalise the routines and adapt them according to the needs of your own child or children. Please note that the routines are not designed to be followed word for word; rather, please think of them as more of a sequence of stages to help guide you and your child as and when you need them. Feel free to add verbal instructions as required.

I always keep verbal instructions as short and succinct as possible for Eddie. This ensures that the essential message does not become lost in unnecessary language and that the instruction is always clearly signposted for him.

I have deliberately included slightly more detail in the first routine on the next page as an example of how the process works for Eddie and me.

Sample Routine: Home to School

- ☐ Wake up Eddie in bed at 0655.

- ☐ Open curtains and look at the sky (comment on the weather).

- ☐ Switch on the radio alarm clock – listen for the 0700 beeps.

- ☐ Snooze for 10 minutes, then 'Time to get up'.

- ☐ Wrap Eddie in his duvet and squeeze him, giving calming deep pressure contact on his neck, shoulders and arms (only include this step if appropriate for your child).

- ☐ Have the clothes for the day laid out and ready (you could do this the night before).

- ☐ Take off pyjamas and put on pants and trousers, perhaps making a game out of throwing each item for him to catch.

- ☐ 'Arms up' – apply deodorant and body spray (only include this step if deodorant/body spray is appropriate for your child).

- ☐ 'Shirt on.'

- ☐ 'Done – time for breakfast.'

- ☐ Go downstairs together for breakfast. As time is critical, supervise breakfast to ensure he goes to school having eaten something nutritious and calorific (see also the Mealtimes routine in Chapter 7).

- ☐ If needed, put on final items of clothing, such as a jumper, cardigan or socks.

- ☐ Telephone rings, signalling the bus is 5 minutes away. Start a 5-minute countdown to leaving the house.

- ☐ Have a countdown of 5, 4, 3, 2, 1 to allow Eddie to finish off whatever he is doing.

- ☐ Say, 'Finish now – time to clean teeth'.

- ☐ 'Shoes on, pack your bag.' He then puts his shoes on, takes off the headphones and iPad, puts them in his rucksack with his packed lunch and home/school book, and zips up his bag. (See also the Packing a School Bag routine in Chapter 5.)

- ☐ Say, 'Get coat' and 'Bye, bye, house' and then walk together to meet the bus.

- ☐ 'Here's the bus.' Eddie gets on the bus. 'Bye, Bye, Mum.' 'Well done, Eddie.'

Chapter 5

Amend this routine to state, for example, 'walking to school' or 'getting in car', depending on your mode of transport.

Always finish the routine with the final task/event, so it's clear to your child that the routine has been completed; praise your child for having completed it.

Although this may seem rigid and formulaic, establishing a structured routine to follow consistently each day not only gets everything done that needs to be done, but can also give your child comfort and lessen any anxiety. Eventually, you may find your child starts to anticipate and jump to the next stage of the routine before you've prompted them; this shows they are on task and retaining the routine, as well as able to follow it.

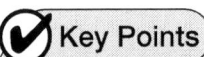 **Key Points**

- Keep language instructive and to a minimum, so as not to overload your child.

- Keep your voice warm and jolly, not hurried and stressed.

- While deep pressure and squeezes can help some children to feel relaxed and help with sensory issues, others may prefer a lighter touch, such as stroking, for reassurance.

- I fling each item of clothing to Eddie, naming it as I do so, which he thinks is funny – especially when his pants land on his head! You may find that peppering routines with humour is a good way of keeping your child on task.

- On non-school days, perhaps leave your child to eat independently.

- If your child HAS to finish something or complete a task as part of their own routine before they leave the house, allow time to do this, but provide a 5, 4, 3, 2, 1 countdown to indicate when this activity has to finish.

- Try to make sure teeth are cleaned in the morning before going to school. This used to be a battle with Eddie, but now we have a routine for this task, embedded as part of the morning and evening/bedtime activities (see Brushing Teeth routine in Chapter 11).

Eddie Story

If you are relying on third-party transport, such as a Local Authority bus or taxi, I can't stress enough the need to be in close communication with the escort or driver. All transport contracts issued by our Local Authority, for example, stipulate that the driver and escort staff must be contactable by mobile phone at all times. We have had so many dramas as a result of us, or other children on the same bus, not being informed of changes or delays. Here are a few examples:

- The bus broke down and no one phoned to let us know; we were waiting for 45 minutes before we found out what the alternative plan would be.

- The escort phoned the wrong house with the 5-minute warning. When she called us, we went to the end of the road to wait, but she was actually arriving at a different child's house. After about 15 minutes, I realised there was a problem, but Eddie wouldn't go back to the house because that wasn't meant to happen; he had left the house to get on the school bus so he needed to get on the school bus.

- The bus that arrived was a different bus and Eddie wouldn't get on it because it wasn't his usual bus (see the following Social Story™).

- The bus that arrived had either a different driver or a different escort. One of the other children refused to get on it because it wasn't the usual driver or escort, which delayed the journey.

Sample Social Story™ for Changes to School Bus or Driver

I go to school on the school bus.

I like going to school on the white and blue school bus.

Sometimes the white and blue bus is broken.

If the white and blue bus is broken, then I need to go on a different bus.

The bus that takes me to school that day might be a different colour.

That is OK because the bus will still take me to school.

It's OK to be sad that the bus is broken.

But I will still get to school on the [different colour/different driver] school bus.

I will be OK on the [different colour/different driver] school bus.

Packing a School Bag

To begin with, it may be that things are just too rushed in the morning to try and delegate the packing of the school bag to your child. But, after a time, involving your child in the routine can be beneficial in terms of time, and help to increase their co-operation and self-awareness. Their starting to take ownership for part of a routine or a task can also have the effect that they will look for ways to do the same with other routines.

Eddie Story

We actually started this routine because Eddie was leaving things behind at school, like his coat and his lunch box or drinks bottle. He was basically too excited about getting to the bus to come home, or too anxious that the bus might leave without him, to check that he had everything with him. The staff at school devised a pictorial check list for him to tick off the items before he left the classroom with his bag. We decided it would be helpful to devise a similar list and use it when he packed his bag in the morning, too, to reinforce this activity on both sides of the school day.

Planning

- Devise the list of what is needed to be stored in the bag (see suggested list in Chapter 3).

- Choose the order in which to pack the items. Stick to a particular order to locate and pack the items.

- Decide at what point in the Home to School routine you will carry out this task. It can be the last thing you do (see the following sample routine) or could be slotted in before you start breakfast, perhaps. The reason we did it at the end was because it worked well as a consecutive but separate routine.

Sample Routine: Packing a School Bag

- ☐ Eddie has always travelled to school on Local Authority transport: the bus comes at the same time every day and, therefore, the arrival of the bus dictates the timing of our routine.

- ☐ 0740 The escort from the bus telephones us to say that the bus will arrive in 5 minutes.

- ☐ Packing the bag is always the final thing we do before we leave the house, after cleaning teeth.

- ☐ We go to the kitchen table, where everything is laid out, together with the list of what is to be packed.

- ☐ We point to each item on the list (these can be ticked off with a pen as you pack them) and then Eddie puts them in the bag.

- ☐ Zip up the bag.

- ☐ Time to go to the bus.

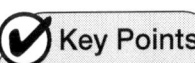

Key Points

Packing a school bag can be complicated by different activities occurring on different days. For example: PE kit needed one day but not every day; wallet/ travel pass for trips out in the community only needed on one day. If this is the case, have a different check list for each day or have an additional items section.

It's preferable to include packing items such as an iPad and headphones in the school bag, as it helps to make sure your child is not distracted by looking at a device, and just going through the motions as they tick off the items and put them in the bag.

We have no idea why, but Eddie wanted to include a hardback Miffy book that had a clock on it. It seemed important to him that he had chosen an item to take, and he insisted on it being the last item to go into his rucksack. This was his contribution to the schedule, and I think it signified he was comfortable with the whole routine.

Flexibility and Routines

It is a good idea to practise not having one of the items to hand so your child has to go and find it, as this will undoubtedly happen at some point: 'Oh dear, no apple juice! Get an apple juice from the cupboard.'

Sabotaging the routine deliberately in this way is a good idea when you have time (and of course only when you have an instant solution, e.g. I knew the apple juice was in the cupboard) and when you think your child can tolerate it without a meltdown. That way they can get used to the routine being disrupted/delayed but then see that it can be sorted.

Coping with disruptions and delays can be difficult but is a necessary skill as they do occur in everyday life. While we are inspiring a clear and consistent framework, we do want to instil a degree of flexibility if required.

Getting Dressed

Getting dressed and undressed is an important life skill for children and is all part of moving towards more independence, when they can select clothes and dress themselves. Learning to get dressed independently can really boost a child's self-confidence and can help speed up the morning routine on a school day.

This also becomes vital once they are at school and need to be able to change in and out of sportswear independently. However, it also involves lots of other quite complicated skills that will also need to be mastered:

- The ability to choose clothing and learn a sequence for dressing.

- Fine motor skills for managing buttons, zips and, perhaps, shoelaces.

- The orientation of the body to pull up clothes and get clothes over the head, as well as co-ordinating front and back and right and left.

- Learning to dress according to the weather and seasons.

If your child is struggling, it might be easier to practise some of the above skills separately rather than while your child is getting dressed. There are some activity puzzles and dressing frames that you can buy to help practise doing up buttons, zips, poppers and shoelaces. You may find that giving your child the opportunity to master the skills before trying to use them for actually getting dressed is helpful.

Issue: Dressing Skills

Goal: This may need to be broken down into stages for different sets of clothes for the weekend:

- clothes for a school day
- outer clothes, such as coat, hat and gloves
- shoes – slip on, Velcro fastened shoes or tying shoelaces
- sportswear
- pyjamas and other nightwear

Eddie Story

From a young age, Eddie couldn't wait to take his nappy and his clothes off at the earliest opportunity. You could tell where he had been by the trail of discarded clothes! This was different at the weekends, when he would happily stay in his cotton pyjamas all day. My husband, on one occasion, delivered Eddie to his Saturday play centre in his shortie pyjamas, thinking it was a shorts and T-shirt combo!

Planning

- Visual aids or a check list are likely to be such useful tools for learning to dress because of the number of items of clothing involved.

- You can also provide visuals to reinforce the sequence. Use your own visuals, photos or symbols, or you can buy them online.

- List the items of clothing your child wears (this will depend on age).

- If you want your child to eventually select clothes independently, also put a picture on drawers or wardrobe doors to indicate where clothes are stored.

- Perhaps start practising at the weekend, when you may have more time than on a school morning.

Sample Routine: Getting Dressed

- ☐ Start by laying out the clothes in the order in which they need to be put on (e.g. pants first, shirt/T-shirt, socks, then trousers/skirt and jumper/sweatshirt/cardigan).

- ☐ Show visuals to reinforce the sequence. (If your child can read, then you could write out a list of clothes, which they can tick off as they choose them and put them on.)

- ☐ Reinforce the item of clothing by pointing out the name.

- ☐ Help to identify the front and back of each item of clothing, for example, the front may have a zip or buttons.

- ☐ Give lots of praise for each item of clothing that is put on correctly.

✅ Key Points

Another tactic is to half put on the item of clothing and leave your child to do the rest.

For example, put their feet in the pants and leave them to pull them up, then put their feet in the trousers and leave them to pull them up, or put the shirt over their head and leave them to put their arms through the sleeves.

We used to play a game of me throwing the item of clothing to Eddie which he somehow caught and then put on.

Stick to easier clothes to begin with, to make it easier, such as tracksuit trousers with an elasticated waist and no zip or buttons, or polo- or T-shirts.

Does your child need to sit down to put on pants or trousers?

Occupational Therapists can provide lots of advice on self-care skills, tailored to your child, if you find that you really are not able to make progress.

As stated earlier, learning to get dressed independently can improve a child's self-confidence and help the morning routine to run more smoothly on a school day, so it really is worth persisting and giving your child plenty of time to practise.

Issues with Clothing

Many children with autism have an issue with clothing, especially if they also have a sensory processing difficulty. So if your child is struggling to wear clothes, potential sensory factors might be something you should consider.

Eddie had issues with clothes from an early age:

- He would try to remove any clothing that was tight around his body.

- He showed a strong preference for wearing baggy shorts.

- Ideally, he would go barefoot, and would immediately remove both shoes and socks as soon as he arrived home.

- He is not keen on long-sleeved clothing – to this day, we have to roll up the sleeves to above his elbows so his forearms are uncovered.

- All labels in clothes had to be cut out with scissors, as they irritated his back or neck.

- Woolly jumpers were too prickly and scratchy for him to wear.

- He can't wear anything with plastic additions or transfers on.

- Eddie also doesn't seem to feel the cold and will happily spend the day in a T-shirt indoors, even when it is winter. We have had to find clothes he really is comfortable in for him to tolerate them. Soft cotton or jersey fabrics and fleecy tracksuit trousers seem to work the best.

Seams on clothes can also cause discomfort for some children, but seamless or seam-free clothes are available to lessen this. Body compression shirts are an

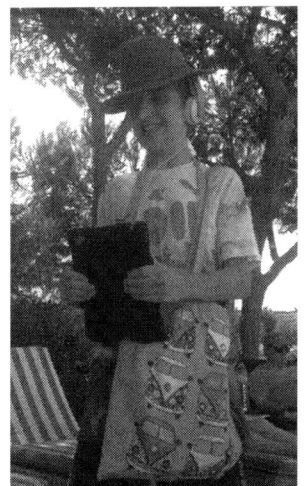

option, too. They are tight-fitting shirts that hug the body and provide sensory input; they don't bunch up on the body, either, as they have some Lycra in them.

Sensory Smart Store is a supplier set up by a mum of an autistic child who had clothing issues for exactly the reasons outlined above and can offer lots of advice from personal experience. You can find the website at www.sensorysmart.co.uk

Dressing on holiday

Toileting

Chapter 5

Children who have autism often have increased difficulties learning toileting skills, for a number of reasons: they may have difficulty in understanding what is expected; they may find the whole toilet environment a sensory trigger due to the smells, noise of the flush, etc.; if they have a restricted diet, they may not have regular bowel movements or they may be constipated; and, also, they may have problems in communicating that they need to use the toilet.

Planning

- Try to be relaxed about toileting, and make the toilet/bathroom a non-threatening place to be.

- Avoid starting toilet training at times of change, such as when you are away on holiday, when you have visitors or when your child is starting nursery.

- Change nappies in the toilet/bathroom so your child associates poo and wee with those rooms.

- Your child may be showing you they are ready to stop wearing nappies when they become fidgety in a nappy or remove it when it's dirty.

- Note: if your child can stay dry for one or two hours that may indicate they are ready to use the toilet and start toilet training.

- Decide whether you want to use a potty or a small-size toilet-training seat with a step-up footstool (which should make it easier for your child to get onto the toilet and get into a comfortable position).

- Use very specific language around toileting, such as 'Let's do a wee now', 'Let's do a poo now'.

- Plan what your reinforcer/reward will be for your child.

- Make sure your child drinks enough fluids.

Timing

Toileting lends itself to being taught as a routine because it involves a sequence of events and actions that happen in the same order each time they use the toilet. For example, your child will always wash their hands after wiping their bottom. But timing is everything and, as a parent, you will most likely be able to tell when your child will need to go to the toilet, even if they haven't recognised that they need to themselves.

Consider the following:

- Children are more likely to poo 20-30 minutes after they have eaten a meal, as eating causes the whole bowel to become more active as food is being digested.

- Try to link going to the toilet to a daily routine, for example, before a meal, after a meal, before leaving the house to go out and before going to bed, so your child gets used to the fact that this is something that happens frequently, not just once a day.

- Put your child on the toilet regularly to see if they need a wee or poo (every two hours or so), but not too often so as to irritate them if they do not need to go.

- Note how often they actually do a wee or poo, to see if there is a pattern emerging.

Sample Routine: Toileting

- ☐ 'It's toilet time.'
- ☐ Go to the toilet.
- ☐ Pull down pants/knickers.
- ☐ Do a wee.
- ☐ Do a poo.
- ☐ Take toilet paper.
- ☐ Wipe (bottom).
- ☐ Pull up clothes.
- ☐ Flush toilet.*
- ☐ Wash hands.
- ☐ Dry hands.
- ☐ Say 'Well done' and reward.

* If your child doesn't like the noise and gushing of the toilet flushing, give them warning or flush the toilet yourself after they have left the area. This step can be added into the routine later, rather than risking the success of the toileting routine because of the anxiety caused by flushing.

If your child doesn't immediately perform a poo or a wee, there are various ways to keep your child on the toilet for a bit longer:

- Play a counting game.

- Give your child a squeezy stress toy to help gently encourage a wee or poo.

- Add food colouring to the toilet water to make it look pretty and, therefore, provide distraction.

- Boys may like to aim at a coloured ping pong ball when peeing, if they are standing up or even sitting down on the toilet.

As mentioned earlier, toileting lends itself to being taught as a routine because it's a sequence of events and actions that are the same every time. For some children with autism, however, just going to the cloakroom/bathroom/toilet cubicle can be difficult. Because of this, as with the Getting Dressed routine, it can work better to break the activity down into stages and reward your child separately for each stage achieved, so that you build up gradually to mastering the whole routine.

One of the products I helped to devise when I owned my shop, SenseToys, was a toilet-training pack, including all the necessary visuals. It is a 10-page, wipe-clean flip book containing pictures backed with hook-and-loop fasteners, providing a visual sequence for the stages of toileting for both boys and girls. It also comes with an 18-page parents' guide written by Dr Eve Fleming, an experienced community paediatrician. The guide has lots of useful information for developing a toileting programme, dealing with toileting problems and night-time toilet training. This pack is available at www.eddiesmum.com

Eddie Story

Quite randomly, and from a fairly early age, Eddie decided that he wanted to squat on the toilet seat to do a poo. Squatting can help to empty the bowel more quickly and completely, without straining. We think that Eddie liked the fact that this made it easier to wipe his bottom. We have, of course, as he has grown larger and heavier, had a few broken toilet seats!

First Stage

- ☐ Time for toilet.
- ☐ Go to toilet.
- ☐ Pulldown pants and sit on the toilet.
- ☐ (Praise and reward if this is achieved).
- ☐ Next time I will try to do a wee/poo.

Second Stage

- ☐ Time for toilet.
- ☐ Go to toilet.
- ☐ Pulldown pants and sit on the toilet, do a wee/poo.
- ☐ (Praise and reward if this is achieved).
- ☐ Next time I will try to wipe my bottom with toilet paper.

Third Stage

- ☐ Time for toilet.
- ☐ Go to toilet.
- ☐ Pulldown pants and sit on the toilet, do a wee/poo.
- ☐ Wipe my bottom with toilet paper.
- ☐ (Praise and reward if this is achieved).
- ☐ Next time I will try to pull up my trousers.

Fourth Stage

- ☐ Time for toilet.
- ☐ Go to toilet.
- ☐ Pulldown pants and sit on the toilet, do a wee/poo.
- ☐ Wipe my bottom and pull up my trousers.
- ☐ (Praise and reward if this is achieved).
- ☐ Next time I will try to flush the toilet.

Chapter 6
Getting Out and About

There will be lots of occasions that necessitate a trip out, such as for a medical appointment or to go on a social outing or to the shops. Some of these trips can be quite stressful for children with autism and, in some cases, are totally intolerable. For example, going for a haircut can be very challenging for children with autism, due to all the sensory and social factors. But over time, with preparation and a personalised set routine, the whole experience can become perfectly comfortable.

So, even though you might have had a bad experience on an outing, which may have led to feelings of negativity and hopelessness that make you dread going out again (we've all been there!), hopefully the ideas in the routines in this section will help you and your child to be able to go out and have enjoyable experiences together.

Going Out in the Car

Fortunately for our family, Eddie has never had a problem with travelling in the car, once he knows where he is going. It's not been the travelling itself that's been the problem, but rather the arriving at a new destination that he hasn't been to before, particularly if it's not where he is expecting to be. So managing his expectations has, and always will be, a priority, in order to help things go smoothly.

If your daily car journey is a school run, you can add the Going out in the Car plan to the Home to School routine.

> ### Eddie Story
>
> One of the biggest problems we had with Eddie was arriving somewhere: even though we had told Eddie where we were going, he might realise he was near somewhere else he wanted to go and, as soon as he was out of the car, would make a run for it! With no thought for traffic or danger, he would bolt out into the road.
>
> This was a huge problem as, when we tried to redirect him to where we were actually meant to be going, he would just flop to the floor in a meltdown.

Planning

Know where you are going and that you will be able to park. The government's Blue Badge scheme enables disabled drivers or passengers to park as close to their destination as possible; we have found this very helpful.

- I usually try not to arrive too early, to lessen the amount of time we need to wait.

- Have a strict rule that seat belts must be fastened up; as Eddie travelled on a school bus from the age of four, this was not a problem for us – he was used to sitting with a seat belt. If your child is resistant to a seatbelt or finds it particularly uncomfortable there are alternative body harnesses you can buy specifically for children and young people with special needs, learning difficulties and/or challenging behaviour (see, for example, www.crelling.com).

- Some children find it very difficult to go on a journey if you don't follow the same route on each occasion. If this is the case, it could be helpful to use a Social Story™ to prepare your child.

- Allow activities such as electronic devices, books, and fidget/sensory toys because these can help to distract and calm your child.

- If you will be travelling to an activity, check that it is going ahead before you leave home – we arrived at the swimming baths once, only to find the pool had been closed due to contamination (I think a child had accidentally pooed in the pool!), so we couldn't swim and had to go straight back home. It was so difficult to try and explain to Eddie why we couldn't swim. We couldn't even go to a different leisure centre, as this was the one Eddie was familiar with and, therefore, was the one he needed to go to. We had no choice but to go home; it was a very miserable afternoon and could have been avoided if I had phoned beforehand.

Going to the Hairdresser

Having a haircut can be difficult for all young children but, for children with autism, there are so many other factors that often need to be overcome. First, the idea of having someone they are not familiar with touching their head and neck, and using sharp scissors or noisy clippers near them, can cause anxiety. There are lots of strong smells in the hairdresser's, with bleach, shampoos and hairspray, which can be overwhelming, as well as lots of noises, such as music playing and hairdryers blaring. Therefore, what can often seem like a nice treat to us, can be quite an ordeal for our children.

Eddie Story

For ages, we went to the hairdressing salon on a busy street. Eddie would sit in his buggy, looking at the buses, taxis and cars as they went by. He wriggled and whooped when vehicles went by and, somehow, the lovely hairdresser managed to take at least some of his hair off without stabbing him with the scissors. Hair went all over him and the buggy, he ate crackers while hair fell on them, and then he had to spit out the hair. It was not a pleasant experience for him, for me or for the hairdresser. But hair grows and it needs to be cut. Eventually, we realised we needed to tackle this situation and find a way to make it more tolerable for everyone.

Planning

- Find a hairdresser willing to cut your child's hair and brief them thoroughly.

- Explain to the hairdresser why the environment may be challenging for your child – noisy hairdryers, strong odours, etc.

- Agree timings – perhaps book the last appointment of the day, when the salon is quieter, or the first one on a weekend.

- Go through the actual sequence of events with your child before going to the hairdresser: don't spring it on them; give them plenty of warning of when the haircut will be happening.

- Maybe take some photos of the salon and borrow one of the capes they use so that it will look familiar to your child.

- Decide on which comforters to take, such as a squeezy sensory toy, fidget toy or a chew toy.

- Phone the salon ahead of your appointment to check they are on schedule – there is nothing worse than sitting around in the salon for 20 minutes, waiting for your hairdresser to finish their previous client.

Sample Routine: Going to the Hairdresser

- ☐ Arrive at the hairdresser's.
- ☐ Coat off.
- ☐ Cape on.
- ☐ Sit at chair – looking in the mirror.
- ☐ Prop up an iPad or device for your child to watch to distract them.
- ☐ At agreed intervals, offer a drink or a chocolate button as a reward.
- ☐ The hairdresser cuts as much hair as they can, while you give lots of praise to your child.
- ☐ When you think your child is getting near to the end of their tolerance level THEN give a 5-minute warning with the blue sand timer or a 3-minute warning with the yellow sand timer – this lets your child and the hairdresser know how much longer they have left.
- ☐ Give lots of praise, say, 'haircut finished' and give them their reward.
- ☐ Once the haircut is finished, it may be easier to make a quick exit from the salon, so your child knows it's over, and clean them up once you are back at home. Otherwise, include cleaning up as part of your routine, staying to brush off the hair or to blow it off with a hairdryer if your child can tolerate the noise.

✔ Key Points

- Ideally have your child sitting on the seat facing the mirror, to make access easier for the hairdresser; sitting on your lap may work initially but eventually your child will get too big.

- Will your child prefer to see what is going on? If so, stand behind them with a mirror so they can see what is happening at the back of their head.

- If your child prefers to be distracted by using a device, looking at an iPad or watching a cartoon, this is fine – as long as they can keep still.

Scissors vs Clippers

Using the clippers is considerably quicker than scissors, as they can cut off more hair in one go – a 25-minute haircut is reduced to about twelve minutes. But, of course, they make quite a loud buzzing sound, and they vibrate, which can be really difficult to tolerate.

So, once you are ready to introduce the clippers, try to help desensitise your child to the threat of the clippers by just offering them and showing them to your child each time you visit the hairdresser. Perhaps hold the clippers near to your child's hand, so they can feel the vibration and hear the buzzing sound, to try to get them used to it.

If you can purchase some clippers for home, then perhaps let your child see someone else having a haircut with the clippers and, therefore, how quick and easy it is – and, importantly, that it doesn't hurt.

Sample Social Story™ for Going to the Hairdresser for a Haircut

The hair on my head grows.

Each day it gets longer.

On [Saturday] I am going to have my hair cut.

I have to go to the hairdresser.

My Mum/Dad will take me.

I might get messy as my hair falls on to me.

But I will be OK.

I might get messy but it will not hurt.

I can look at myself in the mirror and see my hair being cut.

Or I can play with my [add on toy device/activity].

I will be OK.

I will get a big hug from my Mum/Dad.

After cutting my hair, I can go home.

My Mum/Dad will be happy, and I will be able to [eat my chocolate buttons].

Having my hair cut short is OK.

Going Shopping

I have included going shopping as a routine because, while some children may love going to the shops, I have spoken to so many parents who find it an extremely difficult and unpredictable experience.

It can be unpredictable because there are so many triggers that can affect children with autism in busy shops. Also, shopping may be a difficult concept for those with learning difficulties to understand: food doesn't just appear in the fridge or clothes in our drawers, we need to go and buy them from shops. This assumes you don't purchase EVERYTHING online to be delivered to your home!

It can also be difficult because, if you are browsing in shops, there is not a defined end to the activity for the person with you – unless you have specified a timetable or sequence of shops. Therefore, rather like a walk, it can cause anxiety. But shopping is a life skill that, ideally, we want our children to be able to do.

Eddie Story

We have had many negative, unpleasant and upsetting incidents in shops – mostly people staring and pointing and making either snide or judgemental comments. The choice is to either not go to the shops or ignore other people's rude and ignorant comments. There are, of course, people who are very kind and understanding, too.

One of Eddie's biggest triggers in public places was the noise of a child or baby crying and, worse still, he might try to find the child, if they were nearby, and push them to try to stop them crying. So we had to be very vigilant, and Eddie wore ear defenders all the time.

Eddie actually quite liked the supermarket because everything was stacked very neatly in rows; this appealed to his sense of order and love of lining things up or grouping things together. So, as we went round, he would pick any items up from the floor and put them in the right place.

His favourite area was the milk aisle, and he would run up and down in front of the trolleys full of different milk. He usually made his way straight to the milk aisle when we arrived. Although one day there was a man there, who was almost certainly on the spectrum, doing exactly what Eddie wanted to do. They were actually very respectful of each other, without uttering a word, so both were able to enjoy running up and down in front of the milk display. To this day, if we go into a supermarket Eddie will come out with 2 pints of semi-skimmed milk.

Planning

- Try to arrange to go with just one child.

- Choose one shop, such as a supermarket, to buy a defined list of items.

- Try not to take a device, as that is just another thing to keep an eye on.

- Involve your child in making a list of what you will buy, so they can help you select the right items.

- If going to the supermarket is fine, and it is the smaller shops which are the issue, choose a few shops and make up a sequence of the stores you will visit and what you will buy.

- Decide if you will use self-checkouts, as these can be great if your child likes them but cramped and noisy if they don't.

Sample Routine: Going to a Supermarket

- ☐ 'Time to go shopping' – read Social Story.™
- ☐ Arrive at shop.
- ☐ Child sits in/walks by trolley.
- ☐ Look at shopping list.
- ☐ Put items in trolley.
- ☐ Lots of praise and reassurance.
- ☐ Put items on conveyor belt together (if your child enjoys doing this).
- ☐ Pay at checkout.
- ☐ Use sand timer for last few minutes if waiting time is becoming a problem.
- ☐ Lots of praise.
- ☐ Leave supermarket.
- ☐ 'Shopping is done'.
- ☐ Time to go home for reward.

(If you wish to extend the activity, unpack the shopping with your child once home.)

✓ Key Points

- Give your child ear defenders to wear to help soften loud noises.

- If the shop is hot, take off your child's coat while inside to avoid them getting too hot.

- Eddie likes crusty bread, so he would munch through half a baguette while I was shopping.

Sample Social Story™ for Going Shopping

Sometimes I need to go to the shop with Mum/Dad.

Shopping can be fun, as we buy nice/new things.

I will go with Mum/Dad. I will be OK.

I can help Mum/Dad with the shopping.

I can hold the shopping list/tick off the items we buy.

I can put the things we need in the trolley/basket.

I will be helpful, and Mum/Dad will be pleased with me.

Sometimes the shop may not have the item we need.

That is OK. We will be OK not buying that item today.

We can buy that item another day or from another shop.

We must pay for our shopping at the checkout before we leave the shop.

The queue may be long at the checkout, with lots of people.

I will wait. I will be OK waiting with Mum/Dad at the checkout.

I will stay with Mum/Dad at the checkout.

I will not run off.

Running off in the shop is not OK.

Leaving the shop without Mum/Dad is not OK.

Leaving the shop before paying for the shopping is not OK.

Shopping is OK.

I will be OK and when shopping is finished, we can go home/to the park/to the cafe.

Eddie Story

On another occasion, Eddie was on the bus with a carer when they passed a store where we do a lot of shopping together. The bus was a backloading one, with no door at the front, and when it stopped at the traffic lights Eddie jumped off, ran straight across the road – through three lanes of traffic – and into the supermarket. His carer did absolutely the right thing: she ran to the security person at the door and explained that she had lost her autistic child in the store, and the security guard immediately locked down the shop while they found Eddie. He was by the milk, of course, but the carer had not been aware of his passion for the milk aisle! She escorted him out and the shop was re-opened; however, there was a lot of tutting from other shoppers who commented on his 'bad behaviour'. But the important thing was that he was safe.

Going to Buy a Pair of Shoes

I have chosen to cover this situation because, although it was not one that I expected to experience problems with, it was challenging for Eddie from quite an early age. Eddie suddenly became very rigid and inflexible about his shoes: he understood which shoes were his, but not that they were too small or worn out; he simply didn't understand why he needed new shoes; he just wanted to keep the old pair of shoes – 'his shoes'.

Going to a children's shoe shop can be really stressful, as they are often busy with lots of families trying on shoes. You need to wait to have your feet measured. You have to wait for the shoes you have chosen to arrive in your size. You try the shoes on, which aren't your familiar ones. Hopefully, you can get the same style, just in a bigger size, but it's important to get the right fit or you will be back again, buying another pair. We found it was easier if we took a sibling and put them through the same process, so Eddie could see them getting new shoes too. This does, however, prolong the trip – and the waiting around – so may not be possible for everyone.

Planning

1. Identify a shoe shop.
2. Aim to go at a quiet time.
3. Chose a reinforcer to reward your child with.
4. Buy all shoes at once – trainers, school shoes, wellingtons, slippers, etc.
5. Alternatively, have separate trips to reinforce the routine and become more familiar with buying footwear.

Sample Social Story™ for Shopping for New Shoes

I wear shoes every day.

Wearing shoes keeps my feet safe and dry.

I am growing bigger every day.

My shoes do not grow bigger.

When my shoes are too tight, I will need new shoes.

This is OK. I will like my new shoes.

I will go to the shoe shop with Mum/Dad to buy my new shoes.

I will have my feet measured so my new shoes will fit.

I will be OK with having my feet measured.

I will try on new, bigger shoes.

I will be OK with different shoes.

My bigger shoes will fit better.

I will bring my new, bigger shoes home.

I will be OK wearing my new, bigger shoes.

Mum/Dad will be happy that I have new shoes that fit properly.

Going for a Walk

During the lockdowns of 2020 and 2021, and more than ever in this current climate, the link between health and happiness has been recognised; it is widely accepted that people of all ages benefit from time outside, doing some form of exercise, for their physical health and mental wellbeing. So how does this work for children with special needs? Here are some ideas that have come out of my experiences with Eddie, for giving walks a structure, a target and an incentive.

Eddie Story

As Eddie turned 19, we were extremely fortunate to find a wonderful support worker to take him out for exercise sessions at the weekend and on his day off from college. They would go for an exercise session on the machines at the local gym, or cycling sessions in the nearby park or crazy golf at a nearby adventure golf centre. All these activities were enjoyable and beneficial for Eddie, getting him out and about, using up some energy and diverting him from the iPad screen that he so loves! It also helped to build a new relationship for him and to develop camaraderie with his male carer, which is far more appropriate, now he is an adult, than going everywhere with his Mum!

However, with the various restrictions and lockdowns in 2020 and 2021, these activities closed. So we were struggling to get him outside often enough and for any length of time. Eddie's autism makes it difficult for him to understand the point of going for a walk just for the sake of walking and enjoying some time outside, even in the park, on a beach, up a hill or just round town: the restrictions made this doubly challenging. Spectacular views, fresh air or sunny weather seem to hold no enjoyment for Eddie on their own and may actually add to his anxiety and stress levels. I believe this is because he cannot understand walking just for the sake of walking. So we needed to build some structure into the walk for him.

Structuring the Walk

Eddie understands the point of the journeys listed below, as there is usually a reason to go there, a start point and an end point:

- walking to the beach – to go in the sea (this is only possible in the summer because, when we tried this in the autumn, he got upset that we were not all going to swim or board in the sea!)

- walking from the tube station to go to college

- walking to the bus stop to go to the sports centre gym
- walking to the shops to buy food
- walking to the hairdresser's to get his hair cut.

However, he finds walking outside for a break, or as an enjoyable activity, extremely difficult and will frequently express his inability to cope by falling to the ground and rolling around in dismay, even on the wettest grass or muddiest ground. If he is unsure where he is going, even on an outing, he might dash suddenly into a busy road or jump out of the doors on a bus; this is why he needs to have all plans listed for him or made into a Social Story™ that includes reassuring messages of how he will cope and that he will be safe.

As Eddie is too old to go to the park to play on swings or slides now, one idea we had was to devise a check list of landmarks for Eddie to tick off as he went on a circuit walk about town. We used this route several times before varying it, and we avoided going near any of the places he would go with his carer, as he wouldn't understand why he couldn't go in – so no gym or cycling centre.

Sample Route 1

Tick off each place on a small notepad as you go.

- ☐ First fire station.
- ☐ Then Post Office (ideally have a letter to put in the post box).
- ☐ Then past the park.
- ☐ Then to Co-op to shop (have a list of 3 items to buy).
- ☐ Then back home.

Sample Route 2

Tick off each item/place on this list on a small notepad as you spot them.

- ☐ A bus.
- ☐ A zebra crossing.
- ☐ A food shop.
- ☐ A blue car.
- ☐ A church.
- ☐ Then back home.

Going to an Unfamiliar Place

Some time ago, we were able to have a break in the Lake District. Many people would embrace the opportunity for daily walks over the fields, around a lake or even to local waterfalls! What a place to fill the senses with calm and sensory pleasures. Sadly this is not the case for Eddie, for all the reasons discussed previously. So we needed to try and think of ways to get him outside and make sure that, for each walk or bout of exercise, there was a defined destination that could not be disputed.

For the example below, we planned to walk to a set of sandstone caves on a river: a short walk of about two-and-a-half miles, with stone arches to look through at the end.

Set a Goal: Walk to the caves along the river

Clear Structure:

- ☐ Go in car to car park.
- ☐ Put on walking boots.
- ☐ Walk to caves.
- ☐ Stop to throw stones in the river.
- ☐ Walk to caves.
- ☐ Have a photo taken at the caves.

Incentive:

- ☐ At caves eat my Milky Way
- ☐ Then walk straight back to car.
- ☐ Walking finished.
- ☐ In car.
- ☐ Go straight back home.

Other routes we tried:

- Walking over three snowy fields, building a small snow penguin, eating a Kit-Kat, walking home.
- Walking to a local pond, feeding the ducks, having a photo with the ducks, eating a Kit-Kat, walking home.

Another aspect to think about is that as your child gets older there will be a lot of emphasis on independent travel-training. This is tailored by school, college or your Local Authority to give practical help for disabled people to travel by public transport, on foot or by bike. Being able to travel independently can increase your child's autonomy and improve their self-esteem and confidence. Being less reliant on parents and carers to take them to places can lead to more opportunities for them to take part in social and community activities.

Therefore, starting to expose them to different modes of travel and going to different places will help to foster their independence (if that's likely to be a possibility) but also, in the interim, will help any carers or support workers working with your child.

Finally, I should acknowledge the stress going out can cause for us as parents and carers; it can be very challenging and we can only do the best we can. The possibility of a meltdown when you are out and about, especially if you are the only parent on the walk and, therefore, may need to abandon the walk at some point, causing anguish to your other children. Or, sadly, the judgement you may feel from others witnessing the meltdown can often be enough to deter you from going out at all! However, establishing a structure and making the walk like any other routine you might follow can help to lessen the anxiety and reinforce the routine as an achievable one.

Remember: when things go wrong there can be an awful feeling of failure and you may wonder why you bothered, but when it goes right there is a wonderful feeling of achievement. Hopefully, once your routine is established, it will go right more than it will go wrong.

Chapter 7

Food and Eating

Choosing and eating food can be difficult for children with autism. If this isn't a problem you experience with your child then be very grateful that at least this is not an area you need to work on and move to the next chapter!

Very often, people with autism have a restricted range of foods they are willing to eat, due to a whole range of issues. It may not be the flavour of the food that is the issue as much as the texture (too dry or too wet or too lumpy) or the smell of certain foods. Some foods need to be hot, which can be a turn-off, and some children prefer to only eat food of the same colour, or cannot eat foods that have touched each other on the plate. I think it's unfair to refer to these children as 'picky eaters' or 'fussy eaters' as their behaviour is being driven by a completely different set of rules; if they are very young or non-verbal, they cannot explain why they are rejecting the food item, other than by not eating it or having a meltdown. This is why trying to help your child at mealtimes can become quite stressful.

In addition, some children become very rigid about their eating patterns: where they will eat and how they will eat (such as no longer wanting to use cutlery, even if those skills were previously learned). This may be because they feel safe with the foods they know and like and, therefore, are resistant to trying other foods, however often they see other people eating and enjoying them. So often, Eddie's class treat at the end of term has been a trip to McDonald's or KFC. This is not a treat for Eddie, and I have often thought that I must be one of the only parents desperate for their child to like burgers and chips, mostly for the convenience and because he could then join in with meals with his peers. However, like many children with autism, Eddie has specific sensitivities around food:

- He will only eat certain brands, shapes (e.g. of pasta) or colours of food.

- He will only drink from Waitrose apple juice cartons – this creates a problem each time they change the packaging design.

- He will drink a hot chocolate, but only from a reusable cup with a lid, not from a mug.

- Bagels and baguettes are fine, but ordinary toast or bread is not tolerated.

- He will refuse anything mixed together, like curry, lasagne or spaghetti bolognese.

Eddie Story

Very early on, Eddie became food avoidant. The term 'fussy eating' isn't helpful: he wasn't being fussy; he obviously found some foods very offensive and, as a result, was missing out on lots of tasty and nutritious meals because he was unable to tolerate new foods without a lot of help.

I clearly remember the day when Eddie decided he was no longer going to eat food off a spoon or a fork. He was 18 months old and, overnight, he could no longer tolerate a plastic fork or spoon being directed towards his mouth, let alone inside it.

Instead of eating all the foods that his brother ate (rice, pasta, vegetables, baked beans, chicken nuggets, etc.), he was totally uninterested in food and would only eat finger food of a certain texture – hard and crispy (crackers and rice cakes) or sweet and mushy (hot cross buns with fruit in, satsumas and grapes, toasted bagels).

He constantly mouthed his food, especially green grapes, allowing it to work in and out of his mouth in a masticated mess as he explored the texture and taste. This was a very sensory experience for Eddie, not at all about being hungry.

And this presented huge problems, because we then had to concentrate on simply getting calories into our child rather than a healthy balanced diet. Mealtimes became a struggle: trying to post food into his mouth by hand, while he was watching Teletubbies or Thomas the Tank Engine; he would often clamp his lips tightly shut when offered food and, of course, no one wants to force food into someone.

Eddie had no interest in the other people around the dinner table – clearly, the social aspect of mealtimes and the opportunity to interact was something he really disliked. So we decided to feed him on his own, but introduced a 'mealtime buddy' (a machine-washable, knitted hand puppet with teeth); this method had limited success but did result in Eddie managing to eat meaty sausages, melon, broccoli and Yorkshire puddings – a strange assortment, but more calories and, therefore, very worthwhile.

Eddie will still not eat chips, pizza, burgers, sandwiches, pastry and berries: these foods are all a complete no-no.

Introducing New Foods

Your NHS child development team or a nutritionist can give you advice for providing a balanced diet for your child; the sample routine offered here is for introducing new foods, and we are not suggesting the diet your child should follow. This is a strategy for when you find that simply offering a new food isn't enough to get your child to try it. Many children need to be presented with a new food item over 20 times before they will accept it; you should keep offering it, but without exerting pressure that will cause anxiety or become counter-productive.

Planning

- Choose which food to introduce – consider similar flavours or textures to those that your child already likes.

- Once you have had success with introducing new food, move on to a food group that is missing from your child's diet, such as fruit or vegetables or dairy.

- Choose which edible reinforcer food you will offer once your child has tried, licked or eaten the new food. This must be a food your child really likes as it is an enticement and should be something that will be pleasant in their mouth, e.g. orange, melon, etc.

- Do not worry that the concoction of these different foods will make it worse for your child to tolerate, as the well-known, liked food ('the edible reinforcer food') should overshadow the new food.

- Choose which meal you will introduce the food in and stick to using the same mealtime, and not when you are in hurry. The evening meal is perhaps the best time.

- Be prepared to be surprised and don't be influenced by your own food dislikes. You may not like cabbage or spinach, but your child might. We discovered this when Eddie started to munch on the green leaves of a cauliflower we had cooked, as well as eating the cauliflower itself, which then led us to try giving him other leafy greens such as kale.

- Decide from a practical perspective if you will be doing this food introduction as a 1:1 exercise with your child rather than during a family mealtime. This is important as, while you may feel a 1:1 basis is unsociable, it may be more effective and less disruptive to other family members.

- Once you have chosen the new food item to be introduced, do persist with the same food at the next mealtime and at the next – even if it isn't successful the first time – as this regular exposure over a period of time, and increased familiarity with the food, can help your child learn to tolerate it and, eventually, may result in them liking it.

Sample Routine: Introducing a New Food (Broccoli) at Dinner Time

- ☐ Have a large portion of the vegetable in front of you (in this case, broccoli) as well as some small, chopped up pieces of it ready on a separate plate.

- ☐ Chop up small pieces of the reinforcer food (in this example, melon), on the same plate but separated from the new food item.

- ☐ Let your child begin eating their dinner so they are not really, really hungry.

- ☐ Say, 'Time to eat broccoli', and offer a piece of broccoli, either on a spoon or by hand (do not force it into your child's mouth).

- ☐ Give lots of praise if the new food is touched, licked or eaten.

- ☐ Say, 'Time to eat melon', and offer a piece of melon.

- ☐ Repeat, 'Time to eat broccoli', and offer a piece of broccoli.

- ☐ 'Time to eat lovely melon.'

- ☐ More broccoli.

- ☐ More melon.

- ☐ More broccoli.

- ☐ Only let this go on for five or six attempts, as the food will eventually go cold. By then, you will have a good idea if your child likes it or not.

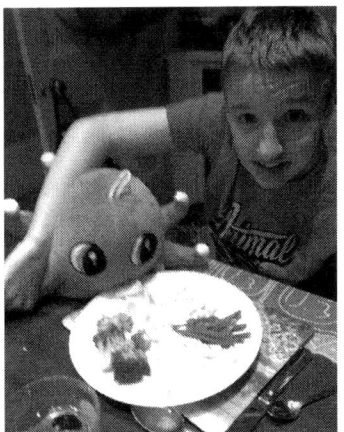

Useful Props

Have a trusted toy or a fiddle toy on the table, especially if your child is non-verbal and they are not interacting with the conversation as everyone else around the table might be.

Use a friendly puppet with a mouth as a 'meal buddy' who tastes the food before your child does. 'Feed' a piece of the

Eddie and his Mealtime Octopus enjoying dinner together

chosen food in the mouth of the puppet, accompanied by lots of 'yum, yum' and happy noises; let your child take turns with the puppet to eat a piece of the new food. If this works, either make sure the puppet is washable or buy a few of them!

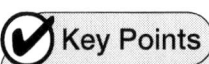 **Key Points**

Don't be tempted to resort to hiding food items that your child has refused inside other food. You may know people who have managed to do this successfully but, if your child has a real issue with food for the reasons we have discussed, this simply won't work and may even make them more averse to trying food they aren't familiar with in future.

Eddie Story

Be careful about hiding medicine in food. This is tricky because obviously you may need your child to take medicine, if it's been prescribed, or they need relief from high temperature, for example. Eddie had been prescribed antibiotics for an ear infection. We broke up the capsules and mixed them in his favourite yoghurt, but the yoghurt was not strong enough to disguise the bitter taste of the antibiotics. He refused to eat the yoghurt – not just that day but for weeks after – and it took another food trial to win him back to eating yoghurt, probably his main source of calcium, again. And it didn't cure the ear infection, so it was a huge step backwards.

Always be ready for something totally random to happen. On a positive note, we actually found out Eddie liked smoked haddock when he took a piece off his sister's plate one mealtime. Without any effort, we had added another food item, rich in calcium and minerals, and he still eats it to this day! Obviously, we didn't want him to routinely take food from other people's plates, but it did encourage us to offer him a bite of our food, in a relaxed informal way, just to see if he would take to it.

Finally and very importantly, if food and eating becomes a serious issue, you should seek specialist help from nutrition professionals. You can find lots of helpful information in the book *Food Refusal and Avoidant Eating in Children, including those with Autism Spectrum Conditions: A Practical Guide for Parents and Professionals* by Gillian Harris and Elizabeth Shea (2018, Jessica Kingsley Publishers).

Routine for Mealtimes

Having a regular pattern of meals, and a structure to mealtimes, is good for many children and especially those with autism, who particularly benefit from consistency.

Planning

- What times suit your family schedule to have your three main meals: breakfast, lunch and dinner?

- Where will the meals take place – in the kitchen or dining area?

- Do you want everyone to sit in the same place? (Does that help or is it likely to form a rigidity that becomes problematic?)

- How long will the meal last? If your child is not used to sitting at the table, build up over several meals, from a really short time – even if it is just 1 minute to begin with – to a longer time. Use sand timers to show how much sitting-at-the-table time is left.

- Split courses – have a sand timer for the length of time to eat the main meal, have a break and a walk around, then come back to the table and set the sand timer again to eat dessert.

Sample Routine: Evening Meal

- ☐ Give a 5-minute warning, using a 5-minute blue sand timer, that dinner will be ready soon and it's time to sit at the table.

- ☐ Wash hands.

- ☐ Sit at the table.

- ☐ Have the schedule in view, showing, if necessary, what foods will be eaten.

- ☐ Point to the foods or have a check list to tick off the foods on your child's plate once eaten.

- ☐ Give lots of praise for food eaten.

- ☐ Once finished, have a break if that's what your child needs – to get up and walk around or play with a toy – but use a sand timer to signal when this break will end; it should only be a short break or having dessert will be forgotten.

- ☐ Go back to sit at the table for fruit or dessert.

- ☐ Again, give lots of praise during the meal – 'Good sitting', 'Good eating' – as appropriate.

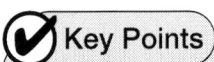 **Key Points**

If possible, avoid allowing your child to walk around with their plate while eating. It's one thing for your child to have issues over what food they eat but if you set clear boundaries as to behaviour at mealtimes, and reinforce them, they will have more time and opportunity to concentrate on trying new foods.

Try to watch out for or be aware of any routine or ritual that your child imposes around eating or at mealtimes, and decide how helpful and necessary it is. Your child wanting to sit in the same seat or eat food in a particular order may not be a problem, but if they insist on it being prepared by the same person, this will become more difficult to accommodate.

Eating Out

If eating and mealtimes are not too challenging for your child, you may want to try eating in a cafe or a restaurant sooner rather than later, so your child becomes familiar with doing this. If your child becomes very resistant to eating out, then it can make life restrictive for you and other members of the family. Transitioning your child to eat somewhere other than in a house or at school involves them transferring skills, such as eating and toileting, to a new environment, as well as all the social factors of meeting up with other people you know or eating with strangers nearby.

On the following page is a Social Story™ we used for going out to the same cafe for a hot chocolate or an omelette.

It helped to sit by the window, so Eddie could see the high street and look at the traffic while he was waiting and/or eating/drinking. The first few times we used the same restaurant and kept our time there to a minimum, but after a while, it was possible to try other places and to stay for a bit longer on each occasion.

Sample Social Story™ for Eating out

Sometimes people like to eat in restaurants or cafes.

I may go and eat in a restaurant or cafe.

I can eat food I like in a restaurant or cafe.

I will be OK in the restaurant or cafe.

I can eat an [omelette, pasta, burger, cake, etc.].

I can choose what I eat.

I might like to try some new foods or drinks.

I will sit down at a table and wait for my food to arrive.

It might be noisy with music or people talking loudly, but that's OK – I will wear my ear defenders.

I can look around or look out of the window or read my book.

Sometimes we have to wait in restaurants or cafes.

I will be OK waiting.

When my food arrives, I will eat my food.

When I have finished eating or drinking, I can go home.

It is OK to eat in restaurants or cafes.

Mum and Dad like restaurants and cafes.

I might like restaurants and cafes and can go again.

A lot will depend on how helpful and supportive the staff in the restaurant are. Luckily, with more awareness of autism nowadays, we have found it easier to find family-friendly restaurants with staff who understand why you need to sit in a particular place or order food without the sauce or ask them to turn the music down. I found it was not worth persisting with a restaurant that wasn't willing to accommodate our needs: it makes it more stressful for everyone and is likely to deter us all from eating out together.

Chapter 8
Helping Out at Home

Lots of young children like to help out around the house – my daughter certainly loved being Mummy's little helper, and it was an extremely enjoyable shared experience. Many children with ASD may also be keen to have a household job, particularly if it is one that they particularly enjoy, such as loading the washing machine, putting the groceries away, feeding a pet or hoovering. Not only is it a wonderful way for them to contribute, but it also helps to build their confidence and self-esteem.

Eddie Story

During the two total lockdown periods due to Covid-19, the biggest change for Eddie was not being able to go to school. Suddenly the entire daily routine and structure was removed from his schedule, and for a reason that he was not really able to understand. He would turn the pages in his diary, only to see all the activities we had planned for those weeks had been crossed out. Missing out on things I had thought he might be pleased not to have to attend, actually seemed to upset him.

Eddie was wholly and totally resistant to any form of home-schooling initially, so we decided to shift the focus to helping out with jobs around the house and garden. These are the areas we covered: cooking, household jobs (e.g. washing, tidying, cleaning, sorting), recycling and gardening. Within a few weeks, Eddie was flourishing with his new home curriculum. This was no substitute for school, but it meant that this period, which ended up being the best part of 6 months, enabled him to both become helpful around the house and to feel that his contribution was valuable and appreciated.

Furthermore, as a result of Eddie helping with these tasks during lockdown, he now is more willing to continue to carry out his household jobs and has added a few more, such as spontaneously restocking the shelf in the bathroom, putting his wet or dirty gym kit in the laundry room and adding items to the shopping list. It really helped his awareness of how and when he could help, and he could feel proud of this.

Cooking

Helping in any way with any part of the cooking process is good:

- deciding what to cook – e.g. cupcakes, pancakes, banana bread
- weighing out/preparing the ingredients
- putting the shopping away after shopping
- putting things away after washing up
- making a sandwich.

Start by giving your child a list with a job that they already do and tick it off as being done by them. You can then add further steps or jobs to the list as they become more familiar.

Household Jobs

There are lots of jobs your child could help with around the house, but it is best to break each chore into separate tasks to be tackled one step at a time.

Changing a bed:
- remove dirty sheets from bed
- put bedding in washing machine
- add washing liquid and fabric conditioner
- dry bedding on airer or in tumble dryer
- put clean sheets back on bed.

Doing laundry:
- put dirty clothes in laundry basket (reinforce this when something gets dirty or at bathtime)
- sort clothes into darks and whites
- put laundry in washing machine
- add washing liquid and fabric conditioner
- dry on airer or in tumble dryer
- fold dry clothes
- put away clothes in the right drawers, or wardrobe, as appropriate.

TIP: to help orientate your child in their bedroom, put labels of items of clothing on drawers, wardrobes or pegs/hooks in your child's bedroom until they are familiar with where they go.

Cleaning and tidying:
- clean a bicycle or trike
- help you to clean your car
- wipe clean and re-arrange food cupboards
- wipe and re-arrange toy cupboards/shelves
- wipe and re-arrange books on a shelf
- empty wastebins.

Around mealtimes:
- lay the table
- clear the table
- put dishes in the sink.

Recycling

Recycling systems vary from one part of the country to another, so you will need to adapt the activities involved in this task to suit the arrangements where you live.

Dealing with the recycling bins in the kitchen:
As before, I would suggest breaking down the activity to its simplest form and then building on the next stage once the task has become familiar.

- As a basic activity, simply take the bins from the kitchen and empty them into the green crates outside. Do this at the same time every day, perhaps after breakfast or the evening meal?
- Label the outside crates 'paper', 'cans', 'plastic' and 'glass'.
- Sort the items for recycling into these categories, placing in the separate labelled crates.
- On the appropriate evening, move the crates outside the gate for the refuse collectors to empty.
- Bring the crates back inside once they have been emptied.

Gardening

Spending time in a garden, whether in your own garden, a relative's or a community garden, can be a wonderful chance to get some much-needed fresh air and provides plenty of opportunities for your child to get involved. Growing plants from seed, watering them and then watching them grow, as well as just spending some time in an area that perhaps has some herbs or a fragrant lavender plant, can be an extremely rewarding and productive experience.

If you are lucky enough to have a garden, or at least some outside space, it might be nice to create a small sensory garden. Try using fragrant herbs, such as lavender, basil and mint. Maybe you could also fill a shallow plant pot with water and find some pebbles that can be plopped into it for splashing, along with a small watering can? Succulent alpine plants that are safe to touch can offer different textures too.

www.glow.co.uk supplies lots of different ideas for the garden, including solar lights, wind chimes and solar wind spinners. They can all help to make the garden a relaxing and visually appealing space to spend time in with your child.

- picking up garden debris, like leaves and twigs, for the green recycling bag

- raking up leaves

- watering plants with a hose or a watering can

- planting sunflower seeds, tomatoes, cress or something that will grow quite rapidly, to see them develop

- making a hanging basket or decorative trough.

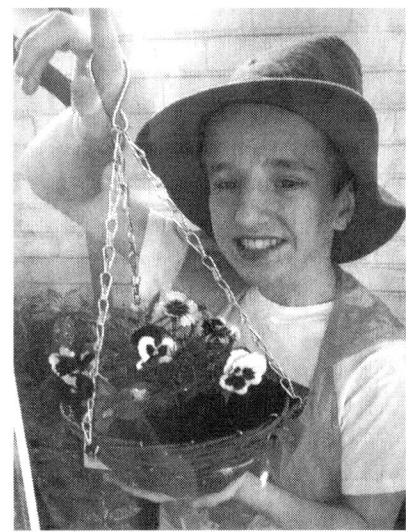

Eddie proudly shows off the hanging basket he made

Chapter 9
Medical Visits

Many children, not only those with autism, feel anxious about going for a medical appointment. This could be because it may involve a physical examination and the child has issues around being touched, but also because often you need to go to the appointment because you aren't feeling well. Quite often the appointments are in very warm, crowded, noisy buildings and they involve a lot of waiting around, so the more we can prepare a child for their appointment, the more likely it is that it will go smoothly.

Going to the Doctor

I have found the key to this is for your GP surgery's receptionist and the doctor you see to have an understanding of autism, how it affects your child and what they can do to accommodate you (rather than thinking you are difficult and want preferential treatment).

Planning

- Speak to your GP surgery's receptionist or go to visit your doctor on your own to politely – but firmly – explain the situation. This will ensure that your surgery's staff understand that this is quite a stressful event for you and your child, and their support and understanding is needed to help it go smoothly.

- Agree timings of when you should arrive and explain that you will need a longer than usual appointment to be able to settle your child. If the surgery can't guarantee that you won't need to wait, ask if you can wait in a side room.

- Use visual supports to explain timings to your child, and/or any procedure they may be having.

- Provide a visual representation of a body that names the body parts, so your child can help to explain where they hurt or see which part of the body the doctor will be looking at.

- Help your child to understand a Pain Measurement Scale, which can be found online and uses faces and colours to indicate if your child is in pain.

- If your child is non-verbal, take their communication book/device/system with you, as they will need to be able to tell you what they want/feel while you are at the appointment; you may discover that, when you are with the doctor, your child can access words and understanding that you hadn't realised they had, because of the situation and how they are feeling.

Eddie Story

One morning, while we were queuing in the doctor's surgery for an appointment, Eddie was toddling up and down the barrier that keeps the queue in a line. Suddenly there was a loud whooping from one of the ladies in the line – Eddie had disappeared inside her furry overcoat. Luckily, she was very understanding!

If your GP surgery usually has toys, in particular one that your child especially likes, make sure they are still there the day before your visit. Eddie had a meltdown before one appointment, when we arrived to find the massive bead frame that he liked had simply vanished – he wanted to search everywhere to see where it had gone!

Sample Routine: Going to See the Doctor

- ☐ 'Time to go to the doctor' – read Social Story™, use visual timetable.
- ☐ Arrive at doctor's surgery.
- ☐ Get a seat in quiet part of waiting room, if possible.
- ☐ Read Social Story™ or look at visuals again for reassurance.
- ☐ Take comforters such as soft toy or sensory toy.
- ☐ Use a sand timer to manage waiting time.
- ☐ Give lots of praise and reassurance – encourage breathing and counting exercises if they help.
- ☐ See the doctor – ask doctor to keep language to a minimum, if that's what your child needs.
- ☐ Give lots of praise and reassurance.
- ☐ Use sand timer for last few minutes if appointment is taking longer than anticipated.
- ☐ Lots more praise.
- ☐ Leave doctor's surgery/go to chemist.
- ☐ Time to go home for reward activity.

Sample Social Story™ for Going to the Doctor

On [day] I will go to see the doctor with Mum/Dad.

We will go in the car and park outside the doctor's building.

I will be OK with Mum/Dad.

The doctor is busy so I will do good waiting for my turn to see the doctor.

I will go into the doctor's room and lie down on the bed.

The doctor will look at my [eyes/nose/ears/tummy].

I will be OK. Mum/Dad can hold my hand.

The doctor may need to use a torch or a mirror.

This is OK. Mum/Dad can hold my hand.

The doctor might need to touch my [eyes/nose/ears/tummy].

This will not hurt.

This is OK. Mum/Dad can hold my hand.

The doctor might take my temperature with a thermometer.

This will not hurt.

The doctor might need to use a tool to look in my ears.

This will not hurt.

This is OK. Mum/Dad can hold my hand.

I will sit on a chair while Mum/Dad talks to the doctor.

I can be brave. Going to the doctor is OK.

If I need medicine, we may need to go to the chemist to get medicine.

I can go to the chemist. That will be OK as medicine will make me feel better.

Then I will go back home.

The doctor is finished.

I did really well.

Remember, as the parent of your child, you will be the one most tuned in to what is best for them, how they can cope, what level of pain they are in and what, if any, medication they will be able to tolerate. You should feel that you can be honest and ask lots of questions so that the doctor understands what will work for your child and what will not work.

Going to the Dentist

There aren't many people who like going to the dentist and, because of the invasive nature of a dental check-up and all the sensory issues that the dentist's room usually presents, it's useful to have a plan for how to help your child cope with it.

Planning

Find a paediatric dentist who is used to dealing with, or ideally specialises in, dealing with children with autism and learning difficulties, and brief them thoroughly.

- Agree timings with the dentist as you won't want to be waiting around too long with your child.

- Decide which comforters and props to bring.

- Prepare your child the day before, using aids such as visuals and timings.

- Go through the actual sequence of events – waiting, wearing dark glasses to shield from the light, etc.

- If using a Social Story™, devise the story and personalise it for your child.

- Perhaps do a role-play practice at home.

- If your child is non-verbal, take their communication book/ device/system with you, so your child will be able to tell you what they want/feel during the appointment.

- Our dentist also agreed to check Pingu's teeth; this was greatly reassuring for Eddie and gave him the confidence to let the dentist look at his own teeth.

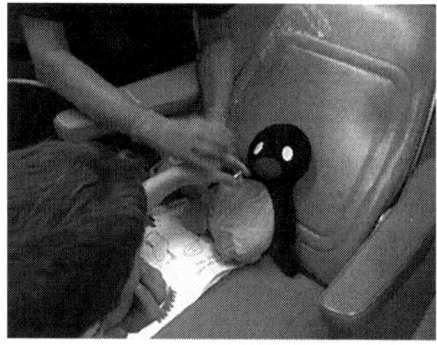

Some fun role play as Eddie supports Pingu having his teeth checked

Sample Social Story™ for Going to the Dentist

Time to go to the dentist.

I will knock on the dentist's door.

I will wait outside on the chair.

The dentist will say, 'Hello, Eddie'.

I will play with some of her toys. She has a bead frame – I like bead frames.

Going to the dentist is OK.

After playing with the toys, I will sit on her big chair.

There will be bright lights in the dentist's room.

I will wear the special dentist glasses.

I will be OK.

I will open my mouth for the dentist.

The dentist will look inside my mouth.

I will keep my mouth open very wide.

I will be OK. Going to the dentist is OK.

The dentist will count my teeth.

The dentist will use a small mirror to look at my teeth.

The dentist will touch my teeth.

The dentist will not hurt me.

I will be OK.

Dentist is finished.

I have a big hug with Mum/Dad.

Well done, Eddie.

I can choose a sticker.

I will go home with Mum/Dad.

Chapter 9

You would read through the Social Story™ the week before the dentist appointment, the day before the appointment, before you go to the appointment and even take it with you to refer to at the dental surgery. It should support everything that happens: what is described in the Social Story™ should match what actually happens at the appointment. This will reassure your child that the Social Story™ is something that can be relied upon.

Going to the Hospital (for an X-ray)

Hopefully, this is not one that you will need to use much, if at all, in your child's life. But if you do for any reason, like we needed to, then this plan might be helpful. It can also be adapted for any other hospital procedure. Going to a hospital differs from going to the dentist or doctor because hospitals are much larger buildings and can be quite scary for an autistic child. There can be the overpowering smell of disinfectant and the glare from bright lights, as well as being around lots of people and waiting in crowded areas often without enough seats.

In addition, you are probably there because of a particular procedure that will require your child to be touched or involves equipment such as blood pressure monitors or X-rays or scans. Even for adults, this can be overwhelming, but doubly so for your child with special needs, who may have little or no understanding of why this is necessary.

As parents we need to stay calm and confident, providing reassurance for our child that everything will go well – while also being prepared for it to not necessarily go to plan.

Planning

- Find out exactly where you will need to go.

- Ask if your child can have the first appointment of the day, so that the hospital will be less crowded.

- Ideally, speak to a receptionist to get any information that you need, such as how long the procedure will take.

- Sometimes the hospital can provide visuals to aid your child's understanding.

- Decide which comforters, fidget toys and reinforcers to use.

- Personalise a Social Story™ for this situation.

- Perhaps do a role-play practice at home if you have some relevant props.

- If your child is non-verbal, take their communication book/device/system with you, so they are able to tell you what they want/feel while you are at the hospital.

Eddie Story

We have had to go to the hospital with Eddie several times for teeth to be removed, as Eddie had too many. We managed to find a video of the admissions procedure, which was helpful in setting the scene for Eddie. The only thing that differed was that the video showed the patient having an identity bracelet on both arms; the admissions nurse was puzzled and said they only usually put one bracelet on. However, to mirror the video and satisfy Eddie, she kindly put one on each of Eddie's arms.

While Eddie was going to be under a general anaesthetic, we took the opportunity of having his teeth covered in a fissure sealant, which helps protect young teeth, and to take blood samples for testing, all in one go.

The following is a sample Social Story™ for having an outpatients X-ray, where you are going for an appointment, not for an operation or overnight stay. X-rays are a vital part of routine dental check-ups, especially as children get older.

The big issue we found with having an X-ray was that Eddie couldn't tolerate the frame they put in your mouth to take the X-ray, so we needed to go to hospital for this procedure. He was also very unhappy about the radiation cape and the large camera that swings around to get close to the cheek.

Having an X-ray is quite a strange experience so, if you can explain and practise beforehand, it should help to prepare your child.

Sample Social Story™ for Going to Hospital for an X-ray of the Mouth

I need to go to the hospital to have an X-ray of my teeth.

An X-ray is a photograph.

I will be OK. It will not hurt.

I will wait for my turn.

I can look at my iPad/device/book.

If I am scared, I can hold Mum/Dad's hand.

When it is time for my X-ray, I will go to the special room.

I will wear a special cape.

I will put a metal board on my right cheek.

The nurse will take a picture using the X-ray machine.

This is OK. I will be OK and it will not hurt.

I will put a metal board on my left cheek.

The nurse will take a picture using the X-ray machine.

This is OK. I will be OK and it will not hurt.

When X-ray is finished, I can leave the hospital.

I will be very good and have the X-ray, and then I can have my treat.

Finally, technology is changing and may vary from dentist to dentist and hospital to hospital; there are helpful videos on the internet, particularly on YouTube, to help show what a particular procedure entails. It is always best to use videos posted from a reliable source, though, such as the NHS, health trusts or charities, or medical universities, to avoid exposing yourself or your child to inaccurate information.

Going for a Vaccination

Whether it's regular vaccinations as part of the routine child health immunisation programme, or the additional Coronavirus vaccinations, jabs can be a struggle for young children, especially those with autism.

When we get our children immunised as babies, they don't have any choice in the matter: they are literally jabbed as we hold them in our arms and comforted by us afterwards.

This gets progressively more difficult as they grow older because they get bigger and stronger; they can also see the needle and realise it's going to hurt, so will more often try and avoid it.

Injections became another common feature of life as we tried to combat Coronavirus. Eddie doesn't have any underlying health conditions, but it was clear we needed to get him vaccinated so he could return to school and his other activities once they resumed.

With the first jab, we got it completely wrong! We assumed we would need to distract and surprise him, so it would all be over before he realised it, but this was totally the wrong approach for him.

I now believe Eddie has quite a high pain threshold, which is not unusual in people with autism. So it wasn't the actual needle going in that was the problem for him, it was a question of when and who was administering the injection. Rather than turning away from it, he actually wanted to see what was happening.

I will lay out the exact sequence of events that occurred when we took Eddie for his third booster vaccination (the culmination of all my experience of vaccinations for Eddie!), to illustrate how much patience, encouragement and repetition on my part and co-operation, patience and reinforcement by the pharmacist/doctor was needed to get us to the point of Eddie allowing the injection.

Planning

- We opted for the first appointment before the pharmacy properly opened so we could take Eddie to school afterwards for the cooking lesson he was looking forward to. That was the reinforcer. However, it might be best to try to get the last appointment of the day so as not to be under the time constraint of other patients waiting to be seen after you.

- The doctor/pharmacist was briefed in no uncertain terms that this was going to be difficult (the first jab had taken 45 minutes). We advised them to keep language to a minimum and use a friendly manner.

Sample Routine: Going for a Vaccination

- ☐ They agreed to do a 'fake jab' on Pingu first and allowed Eddie to go through his ritual of walking around the screen, looking at the clock, walking back to the chair, sitting on the chair and repeating this sequence as many times as he wanted.

- ☐ Eddie kept looking at the clock and I kept calmly reinforcing, 'We need to have jab by 0930, Ed, so we can get to cooking for 10 o'clock', 'Time for jab now, Eddie'.

- ☐ He then came and sat on the chair and touched the injection syringe, but then went away again to repeat his own sequence described above.

- ☐ He came back to the chair, to watch the fake jab on Pingu.

- ☐ More of his ritual of walking around the screen, looking at the clock, walking back to the chair, sitting on the chair.

- ☐ More encouragement given: 'We need to have jab by 0930, Ed, so we can get to cooking for 10 o'clock', 'Time for jab now, Eddie'.

- ☐ Back to the chair, sleeve rolled up, looking at the needle.

- ☐ His ritual of walking around the screen, looking at the clock, walking back to the chair, sitting on the chair was repeated.

- ☐ I gave more encouragement: 'We need to have jab by 0930, Ed, so we can get to cooking for 10 o'clock.'

- ☐ He came back to the chair and this time reached out for the needle, almost 'hand over hand', and allowed the pharmacist to give him the jab while he watched the needle go in.

- ☐ I gave Eddie lots and lots of praise and hugs.

- ☐ Eddie had a photo taken with his Covid card.

- ☐ 'Jab finished now – time to go to school for cooking class.'

Again, this whole process took about 40 minutes. But the co-operation of the pharmacist was key: she didn't bombard Eddie by talking unnecessarily, allowing me to give Eddie the language prompts and encouragement he needed, and to follow and judge by Eddie's lead as to when he was actually ready. By the time we went to have the booster jab, we had got the time down to 30 minutes!

Sample Social Story™ for Going for a Vaccination

I don't like being ill.

Lots of people have been ill with Covid-19.

I have been washing my hands.

I have been wearing a face mask.

But I also need to have a vaccination to stop me being ill.

I will go to the doctor/vaccination centre/pharmacy.

I will sit and watch my Mum/Dad have the vaccination.

I will be OK. Having the vaccination is good. I will be OK.

Mum/Dad will tell me that it hurts a little bit.

Mum/Dad will sit still while she/he has the vaccination.

I will wait for my turn to have the vaccination.

I will watch while I have the vaccination in my arm.

I will sit still.

I will hold my [Pingu toy/comforter].

I will count to three.

I will sit still.

When it is finished, I will be so happy it is over.

I will get my card to say I have had the vaccination.

I will be very pleased/proud.

Mum/Dad will be very pleased with me.

I will sit and eat my [chocolate buttons].

I will wait 15 minutes, then I can LEAVE.

I can read my book/play on my device.

Vaccination finished – I did really well.

Now I can go home/to school.

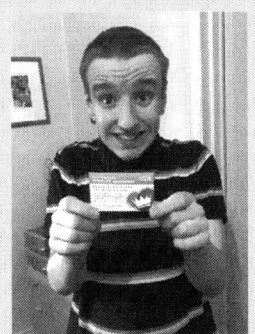

Eddie proudly showing his vaccination card

Chapter 10
Special Events

A nice part of family life is joining in with events and outings with friends and family. These times should be pleasurable, and can often create lasting memories of people we know and places we have been together. While we might find these occasions really enjoyable, for our autistic children they can be rather overwhelming, because every different place we go will require a new set of rules and boundaries that at first are unfamiliar.

In this section, there are ideas and strategies that will hopefully make you feel able to try some of these events and outings; as always, if things do not run smoothly the first time, that doesn't mean your child will never enjoy or tolerate the place or event, and you should not be put off from trying again on another occasion.

We also need to be mindful of how life is for siblings of our autistic child and how we balance what we feel able to do for all our children. There is more about this later, in Chapter 12.

Having a Birthday Party

It is well known that parties and social gatherings are situations that autistic people often find at best difficult or at worst unbearable. Even if it is a party for themselves or a close family member they are often only just about to tolerate the situation and maybe only for a short length of time.

Planning

- Have a really limited number of people the first time your child experiences a party and build up gradually to more guests.

- Perhaps consider a combined party: Eddie's birthday fell in the summer holidays so rather than having a birthday party (as Eddie has no friends) or birthday tea at home, if he was at the Play Centre on his birthday they would arrange balloons, a cake and sing happy birthday to him there.

- Where would your child be comfortable having the party – at home where it would be unusual to have lots of people or in a different party venue?

- Sometimes an activity party, such as tenpin bowling, trampolining or swimming, may be easier than one with party games.

- Having an entertainer or magician might be an option if your child is able to focus and be engaged in this way, but all the child interaction and screaming that would entail could be overwhelming.

- If your child does not show interest in the parcel or presents, cut holes in the wrapping paper so they can get a peek of what is inside.

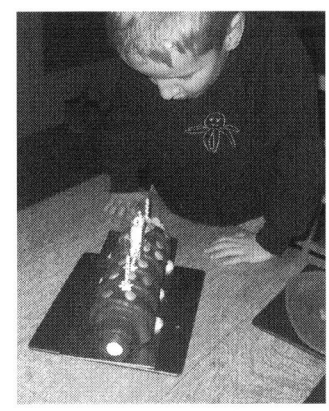

Eddie's birthday cake

- Make sure you have an exit strategy if your child becomes overwhelmed or needs a break.

- I know this is easy to say, but try to keep fuss to a minimum so you are not getting stressed and passing on any anxiety to your child.

Eddie Story

For us it was painfully obvious, very early on, that Eddie was not going to be able to tolerate birthday parties. His second birthday coincided with his sister's christening, so we combined the two occasions as we would already have the family together. The social side of the event was a total disaster.

Eddie couldn't tolerate sitting with the other children at the birthday meal; he kept running off up to his bedroom and bouncing on the bed with his toy squids. If we tried to bring him downstairs, he cried and ran away. He didn't like the food, the chatter or the games. His cousins were upset as they thought they had done something wrong, and we were upset as we felt distraught that Eddie did not want to join in with his own party. For Eddie, he couldn't talk to people, he didn't like the noisy games or the unfamiliar food and he didn't understand getting birthday presents.

STOP – what problem are we trying to solve here?

Trying to go along with a party in the usual format, when this was not what Eddie wanted and was really distressing for everyone. It was particularly unfair on Eddie – after all, it was meant to be his special day? So for quite a few years, we would do very low key celebrations that would involve an activity rather than an actual party.

However, once Eddie was 4 years old, we decided to implement the following Birthday Party programme.

Sample Routine: Practising a Birthday Party

- ☐ Choose a favourite toy as a companion for the party (we used Pingu).
- ☐ Pingu and Eddie would sit on the floor.
- ☐ 'Birthday party time!'
- ☐ Pingu and Eddie would play pass the parcel, with music on very, very quietly in the background, which definitely had to be a song he liked and could tolerate.
- ☐ We would have a small wooden toy cake with candles.
- ☐ We would whisper the 'Happy Birthday' song, not sing it, and certainly not do this loudly.
- ☐ Eddie and Pingu would take turns to blow out the candles.
- ☐ Eddie and Pingu would take turns to cut the cake and serve a slice of cake to each other.
- ☐ Eddie and Pingu would have a dance at the end.
- ☐ The end of party and time to 'go home'.

We held this pretend party with Pingu every week. By the time it came to Eddie's actual birthday, we were able to have his brother and sister sitting on the floor too. We used a real cake, real candles and a real knife. We followed exactly the same routine as the pretend party, not allowing anything unexpected to happen that hadn't been part of the practice party. By the time he was 13, Eddie was lighting the candles with a lighter, cutting the cake himself and tolerating the 'Happy Birthday' song (with ear defenders).

Sample Social Story™ for Going to a Birthday Party

On Saturday, I am going to [Uncle John's] birthday party.

It is a happy day, and my family will be there.

There will be lots of other people there too.

There will be some people I don't know.

It might be noisy, but I will be OK.

I can wear my ear defenders if it gets too noisy.

There will be presents at this party – but they are not mine.

The presents are for [Uncle John] as it's his birthday.

I must not open the presents.

I can join in with the games if I want to.

I can join in with the dancing if I want to.

If I need a break, I just tell Mum/Dad and I can go and sit somewhere quieter with my book/device.

People might sing 'Happy Birthday'.

[Uncle John] will blow out the candles.

I will be able to have some birthday cake if I want it.

At the end of the day, your child's birthday is about celebrating their special day in a way they will enjoy, so they will look forward to the next one.

Going to the Beach

Spending time on the beach with family and friends, exploring rock pools and building sandcastles, should be relaxing, fun and stress-free. However, for an autistic child it can be a very different experience, as a beach offers a huge amount of sensory overload:

- The sea and the sound of the waves, especially if they are crashing on a windy day.

- The sight of the waves as they rumble towards you.

- The salty smell of the sea and the salty spray.

- The sensation of the sand all over your body and between your toes.

- The heat and brightness of the sun.

- The sight of dogs running around.

- The noise of babies crying and other children squealing.

Planning

It may be that a short walk on a beach, just to experience the seaside as a quick visit rather than a day out, might be a good place to start; this can help to avoid your first big day out on the beach going wrong and having to be abandoned because you and your child are both rather overwhelmed by their reaction.

Consider going to a calm, quiet beach to see how your child reacts to the sensory aspects of the seaside.

- If you have more than one child with you, take another adult to help you so that you can concentrate just on your child with special needs.

- Decide that the beach will be a device-free area – no gadgets or phones, as they don't mix with sand and water!

- Define the time you will be there so that your child knows how long you will stay. Perhaps a visual timetable or tick list, like this:

  - first, beach and sea
  - dry off
  - have a snack/lunch
  - play with bucket and spade
  - play in rockpools
  - ice cream time
  - relax in tent (see following point – this was a total hit)
  - time to go home

- Create a safe place. We found out, quite by accident, that Eddie would quickly calm down and stay for quite some time in a pop-up beach tent. It was a major success as it bought us loads more time on the beach while he played with toy cars, slept or just watched what was happening on the beach from the quietness of his tent. (Though, one time, he went running into the wrong tent as he came out of the water, and we had to retrieve him from a tent where a lady had been trying to change!)

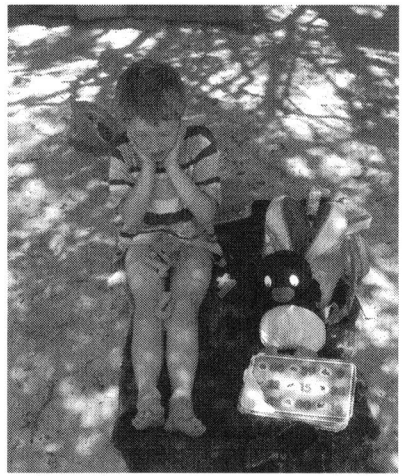

On the beach

- Provide a sun hat and sunglasses to help lessen the brightness of the sun.

- Give plenty of water or juice to drink to help get rid of the taste of salt.

- Plan your next activity so you do have a plan B if you need to leave quickly.

- Recognise the impact on siblings: while it's clear you need to manage the anxieties of your autistic child, you also need to recognise and manage the fact that their sibling(s) may have had a treat cut short and will understandably be upset by that.

Eddie Story

We found that going to the beach in a large family group really helped Eddie, as he watched what the others were doing and this helped him to understand what it was all about. Within 3 years, he was trying to use a body board to surf and really loved it. It also meant that when he had had enough and needed to leave, there would be someone in the group happy to go back to the house with him.

Interestingly, all the things that used to overwhelm him about the beach seem to excite him these days, as over the years he has become used to them. He now hurls himself into the waves, really enjoying them and seems to be totally exhilarated. It's a joy to watch!

Having a Photograph Taken for a Passport

There are many, many reasons why a photograph for a passport application or renewal can be rejected these days. And if you have a child who doesn't really like having his photograph taken, this really can be a challenge. The rules state that if you cannot meet the rules for acceptable passport photos because of a disability, you should give details in your application and send evidence, so maybe that can be your very last resort.

This section is not a routine as such; it's a strategy to effectively achieve a photograph that meets the standard requirements, so you can successfully obtain a passport for your child.

Planning

- Allow plenty of time for this task. Don't leave it to the last minute.

- Practise having photos taken of your child on their own, as you are not allowed to be in the passport photograph with them, however young they are.

- Think about what facial expressions your child likes to see.

- Think about what facial expressions your child can do.

- Obtain some user-friendly expression cards that will help you explain the facial expressions you want your child to do.

Sample Strategy: Having a Photograph Taken for a Passport

☐ Practise having photographs taken – doing different faces.

☐ Use visuals to help your child copy the facial expression, and maybe use a mirror to practise with. Give lots of praise and also have some fun with exaggerating some of the following poses:

- Happy Face – big smiles and laughing

- Angry Face – screwed up face with pursed lips

- Tired/Sleepy Face – yawning and stretching with closed eyes

- Hurt or In-Pain Face – ouch, wrinkling nose and opening mouth

- Monster Face – roaring like a lion or a dragon

- Passport Face – an absolutely still face with eyes open and no expression.

The idea is that all the other faces can be whatever your child wants to do – screwed up faces, lots of expression, hand gestures, eyes open or closed. The emphasis will be on having fun with the other faces but then being very serious and still with Passport Face.

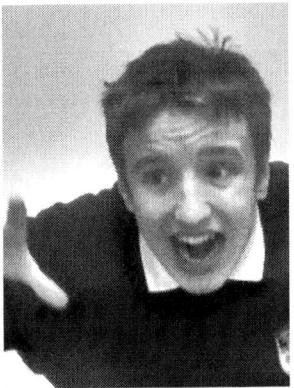
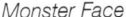

Monster Face

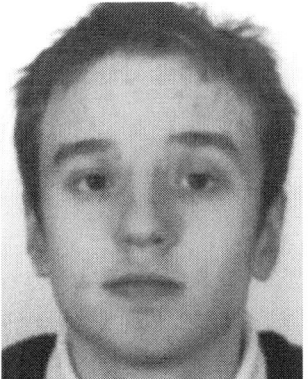

Passport Face

Sample Social Story™ for Having a Passport Photograph Taken

I am going to be travelling soon.

I need to have a passport book to travel.

I need to have a special photograph of me for my passport book.

But I must not smile in the photograph.

I must not laugh in the photograph.

I must not widen my eyes.

I must not close my eyes.

I must not open my mouth.

I must not have anything on my head.

I must have a face showing no emotion.

My face needs to be still.

I will be very good and do my still face.

Mum/Dad will tell me when the photograph is finished.

Then I can smile, laugh and move my face as much as I like.

Eddie Story

Eddie, like many people with autism, had difficulty reading facial expressions and copying faces. He would prefer to avoid looking too much at a face or, if he did look, he would concentrate on one particular feature of the face, such as the hairs of an eyebrow or the dryness of the lips, rather than the whole face or the person whose face he was looking at.

After we had spent a few weeks doing the 'passport photo game', he took a lot more interest in making faces in the mirror and copying our facial expressions and this actually gave us some really positive moments of interaction. This was a delightful, unexpected benefit of needing a passport photo!

Going to an Airport

The good news is that airports have become far more autism friendly in recent years. Some have trained their staff in autism awareness, provide a quiet area and encourage you to ask for assistance if required. Lanyards can also be obtained to allow you to fast track through security queues. We do still, however, have many, many stories of difficulties at the airport, not least because of the very early-morning start or late-night finish, crowds, queuing, waiting and just one process after another that many young or autistic children can't possibly understand the need for. Plus, I am afraid to say, the reactions of other passengers can add to the stress; to have someone judging you and making remarks about you and your child, especially when you are fraught and frazzled yourself, can be quite difficult to deal with.

Eddie Story

On one occasion, we disembarked just before midnight to a really, really long queue in the arrivals hall. There was no way Eddie was going to cope with waiting this time. After 10 minutes or so, he was getting more and more agitated and threw himself on the floor. I managed to find a marshal in a hi-vis jacket and said, pleadingly, 'My son has autism, it's been a really long day, and he can't cope with this great, long queue and the crowds around us. Please can we go to the front?' The marshal reluctantly agreed, but would only allow my husband to accompany Eddie; the rest of us had to stay behind and queue. This rather defeated the object, but at least Eddie and his dad could go through and collect the bags, and Eddie would feel less anxious waiting for us in the car. I felt calmer, but only momentarily, as the woman behind me then declared in a very loud voice to all around us, 'Oh, why don't we all throw ourselves on the floor and get to go to the front of the queue?' To my children's dismay, I squared up to her and asked, 'Would you really like to care for a child with autism 24/7, on the off-chance that half your family could get to the front of a queue in an airport? No, I thought not.'

As I say in the final chapter of this book, over time you grow a thicker skin, you get used to having to explain to people rather than feeling you should apologise to them, and you have the confidence to continue doing what you are doing, or asking for some understanding, in these tricky situations.

The whole journey to your holiday destination can be broken down into three stages:

- getting to the airport
- getting through the airport
- the aeroplane journey.

You can offer a reinforcer at the end of each stage, but the main reinforcer can perhaps be the holiday itself, as you need to get on the aeroplane in order to get to your holiday destination.

Planning

- Check if the airport you are flying from offers provision for people with hidden disabilities. The National Autistic Society has been campaigning for better understanding of the needs of people with autism when they are travelling through airports (for more information, see www.autism.org.uk/what-we-do/news/making-transport-more-inclusive). You can request special assistance – Gatwick North Terminal, for example, now has a sensory room.

- Timings are important, and this is where the airport personnel can particularly help. If they can cut down the queuing time for you by allowing you and your family to go straight to the check-in desk, through passport control and straight through the security checks, this can greatly reduce the time you are waiting around in hot, noisy, crowded areas with strangers.

- Consider all the sensory triggers that could be a problem.

- Consider food and snacks for the journey.

- Be clear you are going to seek all the help you can get from airport personnel to make this journey easier.

Sample Social Story™ for Going to the Airport to Get on an Aeroplane

PHASE 1

I am going away with my family to somewhere that is a long way away.

We can't go on a bus or a train.

The quickest way to get there is on an aeroplane.

We can get on the aeroplane at the airport.

We will get up early to go to the airport.

I am excited to be going on an aeroplane.

I will be OK.

PHASE 2

At the airport, I will have to queue.

I will be OK queuing, as I am happy to be going on an aeroplane.

I will have to show my passport to the official person.

I will have to put my bag through the X-ray machine.

I will have to let the official person search my pockets.

[We have not been able to avoid Eddie being patted down by a security officer.]

Then I will be able to go and wait for the aeroplane.

I will be able to have a snack and a drink.

I will be OK.

I will sit in the waiting area.

I will wait my turn and I will be OK.

PHASE 3

We will be told when it is time to get on the aeroplane.

We will queue to give the airport person our ticket and passport.

We can then walk on to the aeroplane.

We can find our seat and sit down on the aeroplane.

I should put on my seatbelt and relax and play with my [activity/book/device].

If I feel tired, I can sleep on the aeroplane.

The aeroplane ride might be a bit bumpy.

I will wear my seatbelt and I will be OK.

The aeroplane might be noisy, but I will wear my [headphones/ear defenders].

When we are getting ready to land, my ears might hurt.

I can open my mouth wide to stop my ears hurting.

Or I can suck a sweet/swallow a drink to stop my ears hurting.

When the plane is down again, we can get off the aeroplane.

We will need to wait for our bags.

We may need to queue for our bags, but we will be OK.

Going on an aeroplane is fun.

Like visiting the dentist and going for a vaccination, this activity is right up there as a stressful experience for parents of an autistic child, and the awful thing is that it shouldn't be – all you want to do is go on holiday or for a visit, just like everyone else!

I have countless stories I could relate, but I really don't want to put you off going on holiday yourself. And anyway, it didn't stop our family, it just made us find ways to get through it and have the holiday or trip we deserved.

Chapter 11
Evening/Bedtime

I find it very worrying that, left to his own devices, Eddie wouldn't think about washing, cleaning his teeth or showering. He needs to be prompted. In his early teenager years, I did wonder whether all the prompts had actually made the situation worse as he didn't ever need to think about these things for himself. However, given the severity of his learning difficulties, I don't think that is the case. As Eddie has got older, the routines and timings are so embedded that he now often initiates the routine by himself and has a shower.

Bathtime/Showering

Often bathing and showering can be particularly difficult for our children, due to sensory overload from the feel of the water itself, the temperature of the water, the sound of the running water, where the water is coming from (Eddie was very spooked by shower heads), the plug hole and the sound of the water draining away, immersing themselves, washing hair, the scent of the shampoo or bath gels, needing to get dry with a towel, and so on. Although, as adults, we might consider bathtime to be a relaxing and pleasant end to the day, there is simply too much happening for some of our children to be able to process and cope with it.

Bath or Shower?

If you only have either a bath or a shower, then that decision is easy to start with. But, for instance, if you only have a bath in your house, there may still be times – in other people's houses, on holiday, at the swimming pool – where there will only be a shower, so your child will need to be able to tolerate a shower too.

One thing that might help if they are very young, is to get in the bath with your child initially, to help calm them and help them feel safe. This is not ideal and probably not something you will want to continue with for very long. Having other siblings around might help, too, but might also make things a lot more difficult, particularly if they are boisterous, noisy and splashing a lot. Your priority is to get your autistic child bathed and washed, even if this has to be done separately from their siblings to start with.

Planning

- Consider all the sensory issues that may apply to your child.

- Decide on the frequency and timing of bathing – e.g. every day, every other day, morning or evening, before tea or after tea?

- Decide on the sequence of events before bathtime.

- Decide on the sequence of events in the bathroom.

- Which soap or shampoo are you using? Always use the same one so your child is familiar with it.

- How long do you want bathtime to take? Should it be done quickly or slowly?

- What happens after bathtime?

By the time you read this, you are likely to be familiar with which stage of bathing your child is having difficulty with.

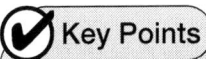

Key Points

- If your child needs distracting, or likes bath toys, then have several to hand – pouring toys, cups, jugs, floating toys or squirty animals are all great. This can be a way of eking out bathtime, or a nice reward for having got the cleaning and washing out of the way. You may even consider washing your child while they are playing, if that works for them.

- Don't wash hair every time you bath them; it's not necessary and is often the most difficult part.

- Try and stay calm, even if things start to get messy, as your child might pick up on your tension.

Sample Routine: Bathtime

- [ ] Prepare the bath to the temperature and depth your child can tolerate. If using bubble bath, make sure it is already in before your child comes into the bathroom.

- [ ] Entice your child into the bath with their favourite bath toys, the 54321 countdown or a sand timer, saying 'Time to get in the bath'.

- [ ] Give your child time to acclimatise.

- [ ] Perhaps pour water from the bath gently over their shoulders to help relax and warm them.

- [ ] Use a soft flannel or sponge to apply soap or gel to wash your child.

- [ ] Wash front, back, underarms and further down the body.

- [ ] Rinse soap off again with gentle pouring of bathwater. Your child may prefer to do this themself.

- [ ] Quickly but gently, massage shampoo into your child's hair and rinse off again by pouring water over the back of their head; have a towel ready to gently mop up any soapy water running down their face.

- [ ] This can be done in about three to five minutes: have your yellow or blue sand timer ready and, if your child has had enough, show them it's now time to get out of the bath.

- [ ] Alternatively, if your child is happy to spend time in the water, this can be a good opportunity to let them soak in the water.

- [ ] Decide where you will be towelling your child dry, e.g. in the bathroom or bedroom. The bathroom might be best as it may be nice and warm from the hot water – dry, apply antiperspirant and put on pyjamas. Use soft, absorbent towels to minimise drying time and rubbing.

- [ ] Put dirty clothes in the laundry basket – 'Bath is finished!'

- [ ] Do not let the water out until your child has left the bathroom, unless they like to watch the bathwater disappear.

- [ ] Give lots of praise to your child and move on to what happens next, e.g. playtime, teeth cleaning, etc.

Chapter 11

Showering

Taking a shower can be a lot quicker and less messy, especially if the shower cubicle is contained by a door. However, there are still sensory issues to consider:

- Is the shower cubicle too small and claustrophobic for your child?

- Is the shower head very powerful? Choose a lighter speed if possible, as shower droplets can feel like bullets raining down on someone.

- Is the shower very noisy? Check the speed of water and power of the water pump.

- If you can find a texture your child can tolerate, is using a sponge helpful?

- Initially, add shower gel to the sponge yourself and build up to your child doing it independently; once the routine is in place, they may well decide to do this on their own as they know it gets the routine over more quickly.

- Do the same with the shampoo – your child may quite quickly prefer to do it themselves, as this puts them in control of the strength of the shower head.

By doing the washing steps in the same order each time you bath or shower your child, they will come to know when they are getting near the end of the routine and this will lessen the need for a sand timer. In fact, one of the bestselling sand timers sold in our shop was the 15-minute purple sand timer for parents with a child who would not get out of the shower, as they had come to enjoy it too much.

Brushing Teeth

Brushing teeth can be a huge problem for autistic children – again, because it is invasive and there are so many sensory and sensitivity issues at play. But oral hygiene is particularly important to help reduce tooth decay and avoid invasive dental treatment. Through regular brushing with high fluoride toothpaste, flossing and a lower sugar diet, hopefully trips to the dentist can be kept to regular check-ups rather than for stressful fillings or other treatments. So it's really important to establish a good routine for the daily brushing of teeth as soon as you can. There are specialist paediatric dentists who can advise and treat autistic children.

Eddie Story

It became clear at age four that Eddie had too many teeth. We were advised that he should have about eight teeth removed – four from the top and four from the bottom of his mouth. There was absolutely no way he could tolerate either the local anaesthetic being put in with a needle or the extractions, so he needed to go to hospital to have the whole procedure done under a general anaesthetic. (See separate Going to the Hospital strategy). While he was asleep, fissure sealants were also brushed onto his teeth to help protect them from decay.

He had to have the same procedure at 9 years of age, under a general anaesthetic at a hospital again, so there was room for his second teeth to come through. While having the anaesthetic was slightly traumatising for him, and the sockets where the teeth had been removed did bleed for a day because he was constantly poking them with his tongue, the result is that the second teeth came through quite neatly and he has nice, even teeth, which makes keeping his teeth clean much easier. Hopefully his wisdom teeth won't necessitate any further hospital treatment.

Planning

- Experiment with different toothbrushes to find one your child can tolerate. Softer bristles will help desensitise teeth and gums to the brushing and make it more tolerable.

- Vibrating toothbrushes are widely available and can give more sensory input, which your child may like.

- Experiment with different toothpastes: some foam up in the mouth, producing a froth that some children find unpleasant; some toothpastes have a very strong mint taste or another flavour, so you can experiment with different brands and tastes. Paediatric dentists often have a range of brands and flavours to recommend.

- If your child is very sensitive to the texture and flavour of toothpaste, you may need to start by having a non-fluoride toothpaste initially.

- Decide where teeth cleaning will take place and make sure the environment is favourable for your child and that everything is to hand to make it happen quickly.

- When to clean teeth in the morning? Have this embedded in your morning routine, ideally after breakfast is finished.

Chapter 11

- When to clean teeth at night – straight after dinner, at bathtime or perhaps immediately before getting into bed as part of a bedtime routine?
- Consider when to introduce flossing.
- Will you clean your child's teeth or let them do it independently?
- Will you use a 2-minute sand timer, for example, to indicate how long brushing needs to last?

Sample Routine: Brushing Teeth

- ☐ At the same time each day (e.g. once breakfast has finished or just before bedtime), say 'Time to clean teeth'.
- ☐ Go into chosen room for toothbrushing.
- ☐ Wet the toothbrush then add toothpaste – 'Time to clean teeth'.
- ☐ Stand behind your child so they can see in the mirror what is happening.
- ☐ Brush top front teeth inside and behind – count 1, 2, 3, 4, 5.
- ☐ Give your child lots of praise.
- ☐ Brush bottom front teeth inside and behind – count 1, 2, 3, 4, 5.
- ☐ Give your child lots of praise.
- ☐ Brush bottom back teeth, all sides and chewing surface – count 1, 2, 3, 4, 5.
- ☐ Give lots of praise again.
- ☐ Brush top back teeth, all sides and chewing surface – count 1, 2, 3, 4, 5.
- ☐ Brush side teeth, all sides – count 1, 2, 3, 4, 5.
- ☐ Give teeth a final brush all round.
- ☐ REWARD: The reward should not be food, obviously, so a sticker chart is usually the best motivational system for teeth cleaning.

Eddie Story

Like everything, the routine you start with will develop and evolve over time as your child grows. We started by cleaning Eddie's teeth in the evenings while he was in the bath playing with his bath toys – this seemed to distract him enough for us to give his teeth a thorough clean. This did involve us standing in the bath sometimes, which his brother and sister found hilarious!

As he got older, he favoured some deep pressure on his jaw and shoulders as we brushed his teeth, standing up, looking in the mirror. He likes to look in the mirror to see what is happening. We eventually mastered rinsing and spitting out once he was about 10 years old.

Sleeping and Bedtime

Establishing a good bedtime routine is a win–win for everyone. If your child sleeps well then hopefully you will sleep well too. I used the same routine for my autistic son as for my other children. Their bedroom was a safe space where they slept every night, all night.

If getting your child with autism to sleep is a struggle every night, this can be really stressful, especially if you have other children; it can mean you have less time and energy for siblings as well as for yourself. It's vitally important that you tackle sleep problems, if you possibly can, and establish a good routine.

Planning

- Sort the bedroom environment first, as this is key to your child being able to relax and will aid restful sleep. This will involve consideration of bedding, lighting and/or nightlights, and comforters.

- Do plenty of activities during the day to wear them out.

- The actual sequence of events before entering the bedroom is important – start your bedtime routine at the same time every night.

- Keep the actual sequence of events in the bedroom consistent.

- It might not be a good idea to allow electronic devices in the bedroom, as they can be overstimulating. The earlier you can incorporate the stage involving switching the device off and leaving it somewhere else into your routine, the better.

- Decide when and how you will withdraw from the room to leave your child to fall asleep on their own.

The bedtime routine should start with a pre-bedtime warning. Maybe in the form of a prompt to clear away toys, switch off devices, have a last drink, etc. This can happen about 15 minutes before going to the bedroom. We have always done this and then gone for a bath, from the bath to clean teeth and then straight to bed. So, actually, the bedtime routine ends up being three routines all in a row.

Ideally, there should be no electronic or computer devices in the bedroom. These need to be switched off and stored away, or left to charge somewhere in a different room, and therefore, this step can be part of the pre-bedtime routine. I appreciate that there will be times when it will be incredibly difficult to stick to this boundary, particularly when your child is ill, for example. However, I do feel that you should try everything you can to persuade your child to stick to this rule. Children, like all of us, need time away from screens, in order to allow them to winddown before sleep. Having the stage of clearing up, getting things ready for the next day, bathtime, storytime and so on, offers a break that allows the body to start releasing melatonin, which is a hormone that naturally encourages the body to sleep.

It's best if the room itself is serene and non-cluttered, but personal to your child so as to be a safe space. Eddie's room had an octopus garden theme because his favourite toy was a furry squid. He had a sea-themed duvet and pillowcase, various toy crabs and lobsters and lots of furry squids, as well as a fleecy blanket with a starfish on it. The room contained a few books and items he had made, but not the usual clutter of a child's bedroom.

Consider lighting: ideally this would be dark or dim, with a bedtime lamp, perhaps, that projects faint images on walls and ceilings, which can help to lull a child to sleep. My children also have glow-in-the-dark stickers on their bedroom ceilings.

Be clear about what is allowed to be in the bed. Eddie went through a phase of sleeping with some maths cubes. I was really worried that these would get swallowed, or he would choke on them, if he fell asleep with them in his mouth. Also, because he wriggled about during the night, they would end up on the floor or behind the bed and we would have to dismantle his room to find the missing cube before he would get dressed in the morning. We needed to break this habit, but the cubes had become some form of ritual comforter that he liked. So, as part of his night-time routine, we played a game of moving them one at a time onto his bedside table. He lined them up neatly in a particular order, of course, but they would still be there the next morning when I went to wake him up. Therefore, for your child to sleep comfortably and not wake up because they are lying on a metal lorry or wooden toy, try to limit what is allowed in their bed and try to include your child in the process of moving these items to a shelf, box or bedside table.

Whenever we went away or stayed elsewhere, a few things from Eddie's room would go with us: his pillowcase, his fleece blanket, a few squids and, of course, Pingu – enough for him to easily identify his safe sleeping space. (See separate routine for Staying Away from Home Overnight.) It would be his safe space, and he would feel reassured and know his place was there, as it is at home. This is a healthy sleep association and, once instilled in your child, will make night-time much easier. It might help to have some photos of your child asleep in their bed, as a reinforcing image of them being safe and happy in bed.

If your child still struggles to settle, you could try putting a weighted blanket on their bed. (See Weighted Therapy Products in Part 1.) These are special blankets that come with weights inside. The weights can be increased depending on the age and size of your child. These are often recommended by occupational therapists for sensory-seeking children, as they help calm their bodies by providing deep pressure support. Rather like being swaddled as a baby to help them feel secure, or being tucked in with sheets and blankets, having a weighted blanket on top of bed covers can foster a feeling of reduced anxiety and calm.

However, weighted blankets should only be used under the guidance of a professional occupational therapist, and usually the weight of the blanket should be no more than 10 per cent of the weight of the child who is sleeping with it.

Chapter 11

Sample Routine: Bedtime

- [ ] Playtime after tea.
- [ ] Playing finishes at 1930.
- [ ] Bathtime.
- [ ] Pyjamas.
- [ ] Clean teeth.
- [ ] Straight to bedroom.
- [ ] Usually a bit of wandering around, maybe some jumping on the bed.
- [ ] Looking for the moon and stars as we close the curtains.
- [ ] Hiding under the duvet.
- [ ] (We didn't have a bedtime story in our routine, as Eddie couldn't follow stories, but this might be where you have your bedtime story, once your child has settled into bed.)
- [ ] Night light on.
- [ ] Say good night.
- [ ] Perhaps one reminder about tomorrow.
- [ ] '[Mummy/Daddy] loves you.'
- [ ] Lights off.
- [ ] Close door.
- [ ] That is it!

Falling Asleep

I think it helps for there to be a final act as part of the routine that signals you will now leave the room. Eddie never wanted to have books read to him at home, so a bedtime story was not an option. If your child likes a story in bed, that could be the final thing you do as part of the routine before you leave the room. Once the story is finished, it's time to go to sleep.

If your child likes and responds to a countdown, that could be another ritual – 5, 4, 3, 2, 1, then lights off and close the door.

For young or really unsettled children, you may be tempted to stay in the room or lie down next to them until they fall asleep. While this might seem helpful in the short term, it can become a habit and thus your child may expect you to be there as they fall asleep as part of the routine. If this is their expectation following illness or a difficult few days, it is possible to gradually phase yourself out of the habit again over a series of consecutive nights:

- First night – sit on the bed
- Second night – sit by the bed
- Third night – sit by the door
- Fourth night – sit outside the room

You may also need to have clear rules about if and when you are willing to return to your child's room. You could promise to pop back in 10 minutes to see if they are OK, but they probably won't have fallen asleep in that time so this may prolong the 'falling asleep phase'. However, you can offer reassurance, say 'see you in the morning' and then close the door. The second time you pop back, you leave it longer than 10 minutes.

Again, if your child wakes in the night and comes to your room, it is usually best to immediately return them to their bed to re-settle them in their own room; try not to let them stay in your bed, as the re-settling should be in their own bedroom to keep establishing and reinforcing this space as their safe place to sleep.

Chapter 11

Staying Away from Home Overnight

At some point, you will probably need to help your child to cope with sleeping somewhere other than in their own bed. This will be because you are staying with friends, or they are staying with another family member overnight, going on holiday, moving house or going to respite care, for example.

Your child may be very excited about this event or they may feel very confused and find the idea quite daunting. For them to adapt to staying away from home overnight, they will need to feel both safe and secure. If you are staying too, that should make it easier for them to make the transition as you will be there to support them.

This section will demonstrate a strategy for making your child feel comfortable sleeping somewhere other than their own home.

Eddie Story

Without fail, on arriving somewhere new, the first thing Eddie would do was search all the rooms to see the layout of the house/apartment and to see where he would be sleeping. So I would always identify where Eddie would be sleeping and put his pillowcase, his fleece blanket and a couple of his toy squids on the bed.

Once he found his room, he knew it would be his safe space just from the presence of a few familiar items, and he would feel reassured and know his place was there. He could then use that area as a quiet space if things got too overwhelming.

If we could, I would obtain photos of the place we were going, and even the room he would be sleeping in, and show them to him in advance, again to foster some familiarity and a sense of things being as he expected them to be.

I don't know why, but he also feels the need to check where all the toilets are, upstairs and downstairs, and this is now part of the settling-in routine that he has established – where he sleeps, where he plays and where the toilets are!

Planning

- Prepare a Social Story™ to explain why you are going to need to sleep away from home.

- Get photos of the bedroom or building where you/your child will be staying.

- Establish how many nights you will be away from home.

- What bedroom items will you take? If your child likes a weighted blanket, for example, take that with you.

- If you have been there before, find a photo of your child in that place or room.

- Be very reassuring about the change rather than overly excited.

- Use a visual schedule to show that bedtime will still be happening but not at home – the sequence of events all still happening as the bedtime routine plays out, should help to lessen uncertainty.

Chapter 11

Sample Routine: Staying Away from Home Overnight

☐ Read through the Social Story™ of what will be happening. The timing of this will depend on whether your child likes lots of warning about a change, and, therefore, needs more time to think about and process the change, or whether you read the Social Story™ as you set up the visual timetable for the next day.

☐ Let your child help you pack their overnight bag and choose what toys/comforters/bedtime story they want to take with them.

☐ When you arrive at the place you will be staying, settle your child in the area they will be spending most of their time.

☐ Set up your child's bedroom with their own bedding.

☐ Take your child up to the bedroom and let them put their toys, pyjamas, nightlight, etc. on the bed so they can see their sleeping place.

☐ Say, 'Here is your bedroom tonight – here is where you will be sleeping'.

☐ Show them where you will be sleeping. Be very reassuring and clear that this is the plan.

☐ Show the visual schedule and, if necessary, read the Social Story™ again.

☐ Get on with your day, then when you start the bathtime/bedtime routine do everything as you would at home, so the only change is the sleeping arrangements.

☐ Praise and encourage your child for doing well.

☐ Save the most praise for after they have managed the overnight sleep. I think it's always good to underplay the thing your child is going to overcome before it happens, then overplay it after they have achieved it, showing excitement and giving lots of praise.

Sample Social Story™ for Staying Away from Home Overnight

On Saturday, I will be going to stay at [Uncle John's house].

I will stay there for one day and one evening.

I will be OK at [Uncle John's house].

I will have fun.

I will have dinner and I will be OK.

I will have a bath/shower and I will be OK.

I will be sleeping in a different bed in [Uncle John's house].

I will take my pillow and my bedding.

I will take my blanket.

I will take my toys.

I will go to bed at my usual bedtime.

I will sleep in the bed at [Uncle John's house] and I will be OK.

And the next day, I will come home, back to my own bed.

My own bed will still be here.

I will be OK and happy sleeping at [Uncle John's house].

This can be amended according to how long you will be away and for any other aspects of being away from home. Clearly, your child will also be eating in a different place, showering/bathing and toileting in different rooms; however, sleeping can often be the most unsettling aspect because your child may be going to bed in an unfamiliar room, either on their own or with other children they are not used to sharing with.

Chapter 11

Chapter 12
YOU and Your Family

Most of this book has been about how you and your family can help your child, so this section focuses on some of the issues that may affect you and why it's important to look after yourself. Again, these views are my personal opinions, based on my own experiences and what I have learned from other parents, and are featured here to try to give you that perspective.

Inability to take care of our own mental and physical health can ultimately result in us becoming exhausted and overwrought, and not being able to meet the needs of our children as well as we usually can. We all know this, but it is easy for it to get lost in the hurly-burly of everyday life, and often our own wellbeing is not prioritised.

Self-care for Parents and Carers

I have met many parents of children with special needs over the years, through running my special educational needs (SEN) toy business, and the common denominators are clear to see. Being a parent of a child with SEN not only involves all the responsibilities you would usually have as a parent, but also requires a huge amount of patience, energy, resourcefulness, determination and resilience: the ability to continually try new things and not to be fazed when you have setbacks. These strengths can be truly remarkable, as in the case of some of the parents I met who had two or three children, all with an ASD diagnosis.

Here are some of the emotions and frustrations I have experienced over the years:

- struggling not to give up because trying to do a new activity has proved too overwhelming

- as one challenge is overcome the next one lies ahead, seeming like an interminable road

- everything feels like a battle as no one seems to understand the needs of your child, or they seem to think they know your child better than you and suggest things that are blatantly unworkable

- the sheer relief when someone 'gets' your child or offers real help

- having to sit quietly and not 'lose it' when other parents are either moaning about or piling pressure on their neurotypical children, and have no comprehension of how difficult it is for you to be able to achieve something, however small, with your child

- stumbling between grief and hopelessness when things go wrong or routines suffer a setback, to then feeling the highs of joyous delight when something, anything, goes right

- constantly having to second guess what Eddie wants or is trying to say, as he cannot make himself understood, and realising how frustrating that must be for him, too.

I think what some people, even close friends, may not appreciate, or perhaps forget, is that it can feel like you are effectively still caring for a small child, even if your child with autism is aged 19. Nothing in their life will happen unless you prompt it, arrange it, supervise it or do it yourself. You may have had children at the same time as your friends but, at some point in the intervening years, their children became independent whereas your child remains totally dependent on you, 24/7.

And, at the back of your mind, there is the issue of who will care for your child in later life. The future hangs over you, offering only uncertainty and more worry. I think it's really important to acknowledge all of these things and to have friends you can talk to about them and to share experiences and concerns.

Sometimes I found it very easy to convince myself that everyone else was doing more than I was, and I felt that they were all probably better at it. It's not a competition. If joining a support group is not for you, it's still really useful to befriend at least one parent with an autistic child of a similar age to yours, so you can chat things through and share ideas and contacts over a cup of tea: they will know exactly what you are going through and their advice and understanding will, in all likelihood, make you feel a bit better and remind you that you are not the only one encountering difficulties.

One of the things I loved about running my exhibition stand at conferences was that teachers and therapists would often have a child in mind when they were sourcing products, and this served as a reminder that there are many committed teachers and assistants out there looking for ideas to help our children. Similarly, parents would often get chatting to each other over a toy or a product, sharing what had worked for their child, or a teacher or therapist would offer some advice on why a particular book or product was good. This definitely helped me to feel less isolated: often these conferences were organised for parents, with all sorts of information on offer and guest speakers to listen to. I couldn't help but feed off the positivity and resilience of the people there.

Every now and then I would meet parents whose child had just received a diagnosis and they were desperate for information, as well as toys and activities their child would be interested in. One of my motivations for writing this book was that, sometimes, I didn't even want to sell these parents anything: I just wanted to share what I had learned over the years that might be useful for their children.

Inadequacy and Guilt

It is true to say that I am often overwhelmed by a feeling of inadequacy. Some days it all feels totally huge and out of control. Why can't Eddie just eat the same as everyone else? Why can't we just get out of the car and go inside the house, without him having to go through his rituals? Should we have had more therapy? Should I be stricter with boundaries, and not allow so much time on the computer?

I found that I had to make a choice and trust my instinct: on the one hand, I wanted to do everything I could to help Eddie, but sometimes I questioned and dreaded the upheaval it would cause. For example, the Gluten-Free, Casein-Free diet is one programme that is suggested to help lessen the effects of autism. We never tried it as, after much research, we felt that the negative nutritional effect on Eddie might outweigh the benefits and that he didn't exhibit the signs of a gluten intolerance, such as diarrhoea. We also didn't get a dog. Trust your instincts to make the decisions that you feel are right for your child.

There are still numerous things that Eddie finds difficult – he is the one who has to deal with not being able to tolerate the things we wish he could like. BUT there is nothing wrong, every now and then, in just admitting to feeling worn out with it all. It's totally fine to have a massive cry, take a deep breath and sleep on it. Then, the next day, get going again because, before you know it, you are staring in wonder at the mind-boggling ability of your child to be so funny or adorable or cheeky, and using that love to bolster your inner strength again for the difficult times.

It's also quite common to feel guilty: that there was something you could have done to avoid the diagnosis or something you did that caused it. For me, these feelings come and go periodically, usually at a time when I am feeling tired and low, and, therefore, more susceptible. It is far better, though, to try and let those feelings go and direct our energies to supporting and enjoying our child.

Acknowledge and Celebrate

Take a moment to acknowledge when things go right. We had a rather torrid time trying to move Eddie on from drinking from a 'sippy' cup/spouted beaker, which are obviously meant for babies and toddlers. Eddie still drank milk from it and loved chewing the spout, so the cups had to be replaced frequently. Eddie was still doing this aged 10 so it was a huge moment of progress when we managed to move him on to drinking from a mug. It had taken a long time and a lot of determination because his milk was a great source of calcium as well as a soother. I felt thrilled, gave myself a big pat on the back and took the time to recognise the importance of this achievement.

There is something special about the way Eddie exudes sheer joy at some very simple things that are totally heart-warming for all of us, too:

- watching endless Thomas the Tank Engine crashes with the same narration
- watching Ronnie O'Sullivan miss a pot for the 99,000th time on YouTube
- plopping small pebbles into a stream
- splashing his sea animals into his bath
- giggling with naughtiness when he has slipped a chocolate Freddo into his pocket without you noticing (but, really, he wants you to know!)
- posting the Social Stories™ that he doesn't like down the back of the radiator
- posting banana skins down the back of the radiator
- splashing in the sea or a swimming pool
- the big smile he gives me when he wakes up in the morning.

Spend time reliving these happy moments, accepting your child with autism as the wonderful, unique and extraordinary person they are, and be proud that you have been able to contribute to that happiness as their mum.

Time for Yourself

For me, this really comes down to wanting a break, to have time to do things without your child, which is totally natural and necessary. But you need to get to a point where you are happy to ask someone or, indeed, you have identified someone who can and will help you to take a break. That person also needs to be confident and capable so that you know your child is safe and happy. For that to happen, especially as your child gets older, you need a support network of people who can help share the load in these ways:

- giving you a few hours off
- taking your child out for a few hours or on an outing
- having your child overnight

- bathing/showering your child and putting them to bed so you can have a free evening.

I found that family and friends and, later on, friends of my other teenage children, were happy to come and 'Eddie-sit' so that we could go out. Eddie has such a well-established evening and bedtime routine that he just needs to be reminded and supervised by a carer. It is also healthy, as well as convenient, that Eddie is happy to be looked after by other people and that he feels safe and secure in the knowledge that we might go out but we will be back.

You really should not feel guilty about arranging some time off – it is so important for your sanity and emotional wellbeing. I found that just having a few hours away helps recharge my batteries so I can face whatever tomorrow brings.

Siblings

Our children with special needs will understandably take up a greater proportion of our time because of their disability and their need for more supervision. This may still be the case, even if there are siblings younger than your child with autism. But it's imperative we give plenty of time to our other children and are aware of when they need extra support too.

I found I needed to acknowledge my other children's feelings and let them be annoyed or angry or confused or embarrassed by Eddie; these reactions are perfectly natural and they needed to be able to express those feelings and have an outlet for them. Once your children have done that, they may feel more connected and invested in helping you to support their autistic sibling too, and giving lots of praise when the sibling is helping you. After all, those are feelings we too, as parents, experience often!

We made a conscious decision to always consider all three of our children when deciding on things such as outings and holidays. We would weigh up whether we should try and include Eddie or whether it was better to let him stay behind with a carer, because actually trying to include him was unfair to him if he really wouldn't enjoy it. The more we did this, the more we got a feel for when it was better to include him.

YES	NO
Crazy Golf	A wedding
Ten Pin Bowling	A Party/Disco
Swimming	A funeral
Water Slides	Skiing
The transport museum	A Pantomime

I think we always found it easier doing things as a group, as Eddie felt he was part of the family and seemed a bit comfier. But there was also the issue of what Eddie was happy to do with us as a family, compared to what he would participate in as part of a school trip. For instance, he was pleased to go to the cinema, Legoland, McDonald's or KFC (though he never ate anything) with school, but he was totally unhappy doing it with me; he would gladly sit through a film for a class trip but wouldn't sit for a Postman Pat show or performance of The Tiger Who Came to Tea with just me.

So it's important to have realistic expectations about what your child is happy to do and with whom. Try not to take it personally if sometimes there are activities that your child is less keen to do with you. Instead, make the most of doing the things he does enjoy doing as a family. We definitely found that there was a 'siblings factor', in that Eddie could be encouraged to do certain things with his brother and sister rather than 1:1, such as swimming, bowling and water slides! Be flexible and open to all possibilities.

Conclusion

To conclude my book, I have included some thoughts from my other children – Oliver, who is two years older than Eddie, and Nicola, 18 months younger than Eddie – on what it was like growing up with a brother with ASD.

Being Eddie's Brother, by Oliver

Growing up with Eddie has been an interesting experience, but it's been a really positive one. I never felt like I was sidelined: I had received my fair share of attention with my own language delay and glue ear operations. Looking back it was odd that we couldn't play together; Eddie always just wanted to do his own thing.

One thing is for certain: it's been a real eye-opener, both for me and for all of my friends who visit our house. I introduce him to them, he acknowledges them with a brief wave and then dives back into whatever he is doing. When I was about 9 years old and started to go to other people's houses, I could see ours was different because we had Eddie. He thinks nothing of streaking through the house with no clothes on and we had all these symbols and timetables to help him learn washing and wiping his bottom. Of course no one minded, they were intrigued! Especially at how well he played snooker.

I got annoyed with him when he showed challenging behaviour in public places like airports, or when we went out for the day, but he couldn't help it. I realise that now.

But everyone loves Eddie – he shows affection and people are happy when he does something well.

Being Eddie's Sister, by Nicola

Even though Eddie is 18 months older than me, he's always felt like my younger brother because of his ASD. From a young age, I was always keen to help my parents with looking after Eddie and I wanted to be involved in his life. Although he prefers to spend time on his own, I used to play games with Eddie and his speech and language therapist every Friday during his sessions when I was in primary school. We would both enjoy this time together and I looked forward to it each week. Especially as I have grown up and no longer live at home, I am so grateful that we had those times together.

One of the most important lessons I've learned from growing up with Eddie is that it helps me put some of my own problems in perspective and stops me feeling stressed about smaller things that actually don't matter that much. I also found my friends would have similar feelings when I introduced them to Eddie – people were never nasty, they were just curious and had a lot of questions to ask me. I never really thought of Eddie as that different until I met my friends' siblings and saw the differences in our home environments.

At times, I did feel that Eddie got more attention, when we were younger and he got to spend more time with my mum, but I would always remember that it was because he just needed more help, and this actually made me very independent from a young age. There were also things he used to do that would annoy me, such as not wanting to wear headphones in the car, or needing to have all of his toys in the back of the car with us. But as we grew up, I began to understand more about why he wanted to do those things and I didn't find them as annoying.

Growing up with Eddie and my other brother has been a very interesting and eye-opening experience. Despite being challenging at times, Eddie is an amazing and loving brother, and he is loved by our whole family.

Being Eddie's Mum, by Lesley: My Social Story™

I am Eddie's Mum.

I love Eddie and he loves me.

Like all people, we have good days and bad days.

The bad days don't last forever.

I will be OK.

The good days I will enjoy and remember and treasure.

I will be OK.

You will be OK too.

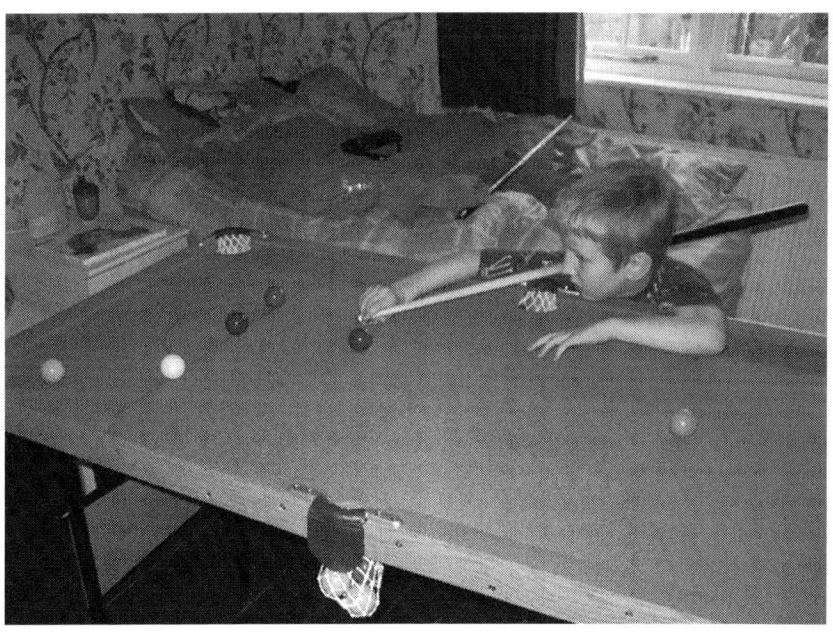

How Eddie holds a snooker cue: he is still awesome at snooker!

Chapter 12

Glossary

AAC device

This stands for Augmentative and Alternative Communication device. It is typically a tablet or a laptop that a person with a speech and language impairment can use to help them to communicate with other people.

Eddie uses a software programme on his iPad which features a menu of words and symbols. When he presses the relevant button, the device says the word he has selected.

Hand-over-hand

Hand-over-hand is a technique for assisting or prompting a child to perform a task by placing your hand over the child's hand and then guiding their hand to perform the task, such as picking up a PECS card or using a toothbrush.

Makaton Signing

Makaton is a unique language programme that uses symbols, signs and speech to enable people to communicate. Hand signing and spoken words are used together to reinforce what is being communicated.

Eddie's specialist nursery taught him to sign the end of day school prayer by the time he was five. It was amazing to watch. Many of the staff at the schools and groups he has attended use Makaton signing.

www.makaton.org

Meltdown

This is when your child has reached the point of being so overwhelmed by a situation that they simply cannot cope. This is typically caused by a previous similarly negative experience or by a succession of events going wrong unexpectedly. Each child will meltdown in their own special way. You may find when they are in full meltdown mode that you are unable to reason with them.

Triggers for Eddie include: being unable to avoid/escape from a crying baby, power cuts, the computer breaking down or an inexplicable, but unavoidable, change of plan (e.g. we have left the house to go swimming but we can't do so as the pool has been closed unexpectedly for some reason).

Non-Verbal

An autistic child who cannot speak may be referred to as non-verbal, even though they may be able to understand others. However, this doesn't mean they cannot or will not be able to communicate. There are several ways to teach children to communicate non-verbally, such as using Makaton (or another sign language), pictures, objects (so children can show what they want), gestures or by moving someone else's hand to the object they want.

Eddie's most telling way of communicating when he was 18 months old was to grab my arm to get me to stand up and then walk me over to the item he wanted. He would let go of my hand when we were in front of the right item. Typically, Eddie would lead me to the TV, if he wanted me to switch it on, his cup, if he wanted a drink, or to a toy on a shelf that he couldn't reach.

PECS

PECS is the Picture Exchange Communication System developed by Andy Bondy and Lori Frost in the USA. It teaches functional communication in a series of six phases, in which a picture is exchanged for a desired item.

www.pecs-unitedkingdom.com

Reinforcer

A reinforcer is an object that is used to reward someone for their positive behaviour. Using the reinforcer/giving the reward straight after a display of positive behaviour helps your child to connect their positive behaviour with the reward.

Although I have often found that sensory toys, such as Koosh balls, work well as reinforcers, you will soon discover what type of reward encourages your child most effectively.

Scripting

Scripting is a regulating behaviour that involves repeating the same words or phrases over and over again. It is also known as 'echolalia'; the person is merely echoing someone else's words, rather than speaking their own thoughts.

There are many scenes from Eddie's favourite TV programmes, such as Noddy and Thomas the Tank Engine, that he repeatedly plays out silently in his head.

Social Stories™

Social Stories™ were originally developed in the USA by Carol Gray. They are used to help children with autism to understand new or challenging social situations.

My Social Stories Book – Carol Gray and Abbie Leigh White, Jessica Kingsley Publishers, 2001

The New Social Story™ Book: Revised and expanded 10th anniversary edition – Carol Gray, Jessica Kingsley Publishers, 2010

www.carolgraysocialstories.com

Stimming

Stimming is short for 'self-stimulation' and includes any number of repetitive behaviours, such as hand-flapping, jumping and fiddling.

Eddie's most common stim is when he holds something next to his face (it could just be his fist) and then waves it about so he can see it both from the side of and in front of his face.

Triad of Impairments

The triad of impairments is a cluster of impairments involving social interaction, communication and imagination. The consequent repetitive pattern of behaviour is the common thread connecting autistic disorders.

The Autistic Spectrum: A guide for parents and professionals – Lorna Wing

Robinson / 240 pp / 2003

Trigger

A trigger (or, sometimes, multiple triggers) causes your child to feel overwhelmed by their environment to the point of being unable to cope. The trigger can be something physical or a memory of a negative experience.

Visuals/Visual Prompts

Many autistic children are visual learners. So, by using a photograph, symbol, picture or Makaton sign at the same time as issuing a verbal instruction, you are helping to support what you are saying to your child.

As the visual prompt is itself a concrete object, the child is aware of it longer than they would be if the word was simply spoken to them. What's more, as the child becomes more familiar with the same visuals appearing in routines and instructions, they will consequently find it quicker and easier to understand what you say.

Eddie often pauses before he responds to an instruction, as if he is taking longer to process what has been said or to understand the symbol or sign that has been placed in front of him. We always give him plenty of time to show he has understood before we repeat the instruction, which ensures we don't interrupt his focus.